THE LEARNING HEALTH SYSTEM SERIES

The State of the U.S. Biomedical and Health Research Enterprise

Strategies for Achieving a Healthier America

Melissa H. Laitner, Audrey M. Huang, and Shannon Takala-Harrison, *Editors*

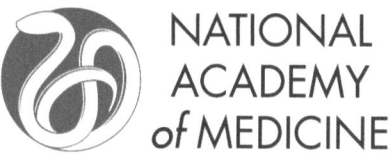

WASHINGTON, DC
NAM.EDU

**NATIONAL
ACADEMIES
PRESS**
Washington, DC

NATIONAL ACADEMIES PRESS   500 Fifth Street, NW   Washington, DC 20001

This publication was initiated and funded by the National Academy of Medicine (NAM). It has undergone peer review according to procedures established by the NAM. Publication by the NAM signifies that it is the product of a carefully considered process and is a contribution worthy of public attention but does not constitute an endorsement of conclusions and recommendations by the NAM. The views presented in this publication are those of individual contributors and do not represent formal consensus positions of the authors' organizations; the NAM; or the National Academies of Sciences, Engineering, and Medicine.

International Standard Book Number-13: 978-0-309-71666-6
International Standard Book Number-10: 0-309-71666-7
Digital Object Identifier: https://doi.org/10.17226/27588

Copyright 2024 by the National Academy of Sciences. National Academies of Sciences, Engineering, and Medicine and National Academies Press and the graphical logos for each are all trademarks of the National Academy of Sciences. All rights reserved.

Printed in the United States of America.

Suggested citation: National Academy of Medicine. 2024. *The State of the U.S. Biomedical and Health Research Enterprise: Strategies for Achieving a Healthier America.* M. H. Laitner, A. M. Huang, and S. Takala-Harrison, editors. NAM Special Publication. Washington, DC: The National Academies Press. https://doi.org/10.17226/27588.

*"Knowing is not enough; we must apply.
Willing is not enough; we must do"*
—GOETHE

LEADERSHIP
INNOVATION
IMPACT

for a healthier future

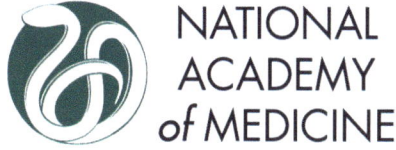

NATIONAL
ACADEMY
of MEDICINE

ABOUT THE NATIONAL ACADEMY OF MEDICINE

The **National Academy of Medicine** is one of three Academies constituting the National Academies of Sciences, Engineering, and Medicine (the National Academies). The National Academies provide independent, objective analysis and advice to the nation and conduct other activities to solve complex problems and inform public policy decisions. The National Academies also encourage education and research, recognize outstanding contributions to knowledge, and increase public understanding in matters of science, engineering, and medicine.

The **National Academy of Sciences** was established in 1863 by an Act of Congress, signed by President Lincoln, as a private, nongovernmental institution to advise the nation on issues related to science and technology. Members are elected by their peers for outstanding contributions to research. Dr. Marcia McNutt is president.

The **National Academy of Engineering** was established in 1964 under the charter of the National Academy of Sciences to bring the practices of engineering to advising the nation. Members are elected by their peers for extraordinary contributions to engineering. Dr. John L. Anderson is president.

The **National Academy of Medicine** (formerly the Institute of Medicine) was established in 1970 under the charter of the National Academy of Sciences to advise the nation on issues of health, health care, and biomedical science and technology. Members are elected by their peers for distinguished contributions to medicine and health. Dr. Victor J. Dzau is president.

Learn more about the National Academy of Medicine at NAM.edu.

THE STATE OF THE U.S. BIOMEDICAL AND HEALTH RESEARCH ENTERPRISE

AUTHOR GROUP

E. ALBERT REECE (*Chair*), University of Maryland School of Medicine
JEFFREY R. BALSER (*Sub-Group Chair*), Vanderbilt University Medical Center
DIANE E. GRIFFIN (*Sub-Group Chair*), Johns Hopkins Bloomberg School of Public Health
KIRSTEN BIBBINS-DOMINGO, University of California, San Francisco; *Journal of the American Medical Association*
VICTOR J. DZAU, National Academy of Medicine
KAFUI DZIRASA, Duke University Medical Center
CLAIRE M. FRASER, University of Maryland School of Medicine
LINDA P. FRIED, Columbia University Mailman School of Public Health
ANN KURTH, The New York Academy of Medicine
SUDIP PARIKH, American Association for the Advancement of Science
RANDALL RUTTA, National Health Council
MARY WOOLLEY, Research!America
KEITH YAMAMOTO, University of California, San Francisco
ELIAS ZERHOUNI, Johns Hopkins University; Opko Health
HUDA Y. ZOGHBI, Baylor College of Medicine

Project Staff

AUDREY M. HUANG, University of Maryland School of Medicine
MELISSA H. LAITNER, National Academy of Medicine
SHANNON TAKALA-HARRISON, University of Maryland School of Medicine

CONSULTATIVE EXPERTS

The author group would like to express its sincere gratitude to the following experts, who were called upon to share their views on the past, present, and future state of the U.S. biomedical research enterprise for this publication. Their insights and knowledge have informed the final form of this publication.

NORMAN R. AUGUSTINE, Lockheed Martin Corporation (retired) and former Undersecretary of the Army
ROY BLUNT, U.S. Senator (R), Missouri
DANIELLE CARNIVAL, White House Office of Science and Technology Policy
FRANCIS S. COLLINS, National Institutes of Health
ROBERT W. CONN, University of California, San Diego
HARVEY V. FINEBERG, Gordon and Betty Moore Foundation
JAMES FLYNN, Deerfield Management Company
MARIA FREIRE, Foundation for the National Institutes of Health
DAVID WHOLLEY, Foundation for the National Institutes of Health (retired)

REVIEWERS

This publication has undergone peer review according to procedures established by the National Academy of Medicine (NAM). As an NAM Special Publication, it is the product of a carefully considered and systematic process and has the approval of the NAM Council. It is not a consensus study of the National Academies of Sciences, Engineering, and Medicine, and does not necessarily represent positions of the individual authors' organizations.

The author group thanks the following individuals for their review of this report:

NORMAN R. AUGUSTINE, Lockheed Martin Corporation (retired) and former Undersecretary of the Army
HARVEY V. FINEBERG, Gordon and Betty Moore Foundation
ANNA GREKA, Brigham and Women's Hospital
RALPH SNYDERMAN, Duke University School of Medicine
SOHAIL TAVAZOIE, The Rockefeller University

The reviewers listed above provided many constructive comments and suggestions, but they were not asked to endorse the content of the Special Publication and did not see the final draft before it was published.

Review of this publication was overseen by **GILBERT S. OMENN,** University of Michigan Medical School. Responsibility for the final content rests entirely with the author group and the National Academy of Medicine.

CONTENTS

Acronyms and Abbreviations xv

Executive Summary 1

1 Introduction 13

2 A Strategic and Coordinated Approach to the U.S. Biomedical Research Enterprise. 31

3 Streamlined, Coordinated, and Increasingly Impactful Funding 57

4 A Renewed Focus on Health Equity 67

5 The Need for Federal Coordination and Use of Convergence Science. 81

6 A 21st-Century Workforce for the U.S. Biomedical Research Enterprise of the Future 89

7 A Renewed and Revitalized U.S. Biomedical Research Enterprise Is Possible 101

References. 105

BOXES, FIGURES, AND TABLE

BOXES

1-1 Definitions of Types of Research Included in the U.S. Biomedical Research Enterprise, 14

2-1 National Agenda Setting Example 1: Singapore, 51
2-2 National Agenda Setting Example 2: China, 52
2-3 National Agenda Setting Example 3: European Union, 53

FIGURES

1-1 Top 10 leading causes of death in the United States, by sex, 2019 and 2020, 15
1-2 National Institutes of Health funding by institute, 1999–2021, 16
1-3 Cancer incidence and mortality in the United States, 1999–2021, 17
1-4 National Institutes of Health funding by year, 22
1-5 Future state of the U.S. biomedical research enterprise, 27

2-1 National Institutes of Health spending on basic and applied research, 2003–2022, 33
2-2 Life expectancy at birth and age 65, by sex: United States, 2021 and 2022, 37
2-3 Maternal mortality rate by race and Hispanic origin: United States, 2021 and 2022, 38
2-4 Age-adjusted suicide rates by sex: United States, 2001–2021, 41
2-5 U.S. deaths due to dementias, 42
2-6 American confidence in scientists falls, 45
2-7 Trust in science varies among groups, 46

2-8 Basic science research expenditures (% gross domestic product) by country, 2000–2021, 50

3-1 Gross expenditures on research and development by country, in terms of % gross domestic product, 2000–2021, 58
3-2 Basic science research expenditures (% gross domestic product) by country, 2000–2021, 59
3-3 Current state of the U.S. biomedical research enterprise, 64

4-1 Prostate cancer: Age-adjusted rate of new cases per 10,000 men by race/ethnicity, 69
4-2 Female breast cancer: Age-adjusted death rate per 100,000 women by race/ethnicity, 70
4-3 Estimated HIV infections in the United States by region, 2021, 71

6-1 Number of U.S. trainees by career stage, 1979–2019, 90
6-2 U.S. postdoctorate recipients, by broad field, 2001 and 2021, 92
6-3 Median annual salary of doctorate recipients with definite commitments in the United States, by position type and broad field, 2021, 93

7-1 Current state of the U.S. biomedical research enterprise, 102
7-2 Future state of the U.S. biomedical research enterprise, 103

TABLE

2-1 Health Conditions Impacting Women and Men in the United States, 2022, 37

ACRONYMS AND ABBREVIATIONS

AIDS	acquired immunodeficiency syndrome
AMP	Accelerating Medicines Partnership
COVID-19	coronavirus disease 2019
FDA	U.S. Food and Drug Administration
FNIH	Foundation for the National Institutes of Health
GDP	gross domestic product
GHIT	Global Health Innovative Technology Fund
HGP	Human Genome Project
HIV	human immunodeficiency virus
LN	lupus nephritis
MLP	Medium- and Long-Term Plan for the Development of Science and Technology
MSI	minority-serving institution
NCI	National Cancer Institute
NHLBI	National Heart, Lung, and Blood Institute
NIAID	National Institute of Allergy and Infectious Diseases
NIDDK	National Institute of Diabetes and Digestive and Kidney Diseases
NIH	National Institutes of Health
NSF	National Science Foundation
OMB	Office of Management and Budget
OSRD	Office of Scientific Research and Development

OWS	Operation Warp Speed
PPP	public–private partnership
R&D	research and development
WHO	World Health Organization

EXECUTIVE SUMMARY[1]

The U.S. biomedical research enterprise—including discovery and translational research conducted by the federal government, pharmaceutical industry, health care, and public health—contributes significantly to America's health and economy. It supports scientific progress nationally and globally, demonstrated by the large number of American-born and -trained scientists who have received the Nobel Prize and have made breakthrough achievements recognized by other accolades. Five of the 10 largest pharmaceutical companies are based in the United States, and America provides many talented global scholars with advanced biomedical training every year. Many international scientists who train in the United States remain in the country and contribute to growing America's knowledge capital and gross domestic product (GDP)—further strengthening the U.S. biomedical research enterprise.

Despite these many positives, the biomedical research enterprise, in its current state, is not achieving all it can. The structure of the enterprise, established in the early 1940s, has not significantly changed since then. It has achieved much in the past 80 years, including reducing cancer mortality, developing medications to treat and prevent HIV/AIDS, sequencing the human genome, and developing and distributing vaccines that helped quell the COVID-19 pandemic—but the challenges facing Americans and, therefore, the enterprise have changed.

First, the health threats causing the highest levels of morbidity and mortality for Americans are increasingly complex, intertwined, and connected to the social determinants of health. These health threats are also almost unilaterally disproportionately impacting minoritized populations, resulting in inexcusable health inequities. For example, within the United States, maternal mortality rates for non-Hispanic Black women are 3.0 times that of Hispanic women and 2.5 times that of White women. Therefore, a single treatment, drug, or diagnostic

---

[1] This Executive Summary does not include references. Citations for the discussion presented in the Executive Summary appear in the subsequent chapters.

will not be able to solve these health problems. A coordinated, transdisciplinary approach is necessary to understand, intervene, and alleviate these diseases—and the current structure of the U.S. biomedical research enterprise struggles to facilitate and fund such convergence science. The enterprise has also never explicitly focused on health equity, and the time for improving the health of *all* Americans is well overdue.

Second, America's peer nations are beginning to invest more and more of their own GDP and person-power into biomedical research while America's investments have remained relatively flat for the past two decades. These peer nations are also developing, implementing, and utilizing national-level strategic plans to guide their investments and areas of focus. The United States has long held a leadership position in biomedical research, but a lack of high-level national coordination results in inconsistent emphasis and growth. This lack of focus will likely put the United States at a disadvantage compared to its peer nations when health challenges are only growing.

Third, structural issues are standing in the way of the enterprise's utmost efficiency and effectiveness—two of which are a lagging workforce and fragmented funding. The U.S. biomedical enterprise would not exist without the scientists, scholars, and related personnel who conduct and support the research that leads to breakthroughs, therapies, and diagnostics. However, the enterprise is not financially competitive when compared to industry and academia, female scientists and those from minoritized backgrounds compose an unacceptably small portion of the workforce, and international scholars who earn their degrees in America are increasingly exiting the U.S. biomedical workforce for employment elsewhere. Although the federal government drives most of America's biomedical research funding, increasingly large contributions from industry, venture capital, and philanthropy bring conflicting agendas that can result in research focused on what is profitable rather than what is beneficial for most Americans.

Now is the time to take bold steps to structurally improve the U.S. biomedical research enterprise, implement efficiencies, increase the use of convergence science, and break down silos. Without these efforts, America risks harming the nation's health and economy.

This National Academy of Medicine (NAM) Special Publication addresses each of these barriers in turn, spending a chapter focusing on the history and current challenges associated with a specific barrier and then proposing actions to address and eliminate it. This Special Publication aims to provide a roadmap for reimagining and reinvigorating the U.S. biomedical research enterprise before a time of dire crisis when all Americans and the world need it to be working at its full efficiency.

AUTHOR GROUP

The NAM appointed a committee to author this Special Publication composed of NAM members and other leaders who are dedicated to health and medical research, its promise, and its future. They have expertise in medicine, nursing, public health, population science, patient advocacy, basic science, academic leadership, education, policy, pharmaceuticals, federal government, and science advocacy. The authors met over a year and reviewed the nation's progress in health and medical research since 1999 with a focus on its current state. They then developed and proposed solutions to ensure that future generations can reap the benefits of a nation that is an innovative leader in health science research.

APPROACH AND METHODOLOGY

The authors reviewed trends over time—including past, current, and growing health challenges, the research funding dedicated to select conditions, and associated mortality and incidence—using publicly available data and focusing primarily on 2000 to today. The authors also interviewed 10 leaders and experts in biomedical research, federal government, philanthropy, and venture capital funds to understand their experience since 2000 and where they believe the U.S. biomedical research enterprise needs attention. The data presented in this Special Publication and the input collected from the 10 interviews served as the basis for 9 months of analysis, discussion, and review, culminating in a hybrid retreat to formulate this Special Publication's priorities for action.

PRIORITIES FOR A RENEWED AND REVITALIZED U.S. BIOMEDICAL RESEARCH ENTERPRISE

Biomedical Research Enterprise Advisory Body and National Strategic Vision

The U.S. biomedical research enterprise is a large and complex entity composed of many actors and serving many agendas. These often conflicting and numerous prerogatives and stakeholders result in a fragmented approach to prioritization and funding that may elevate areas of focus other than the emerging needs of the American people and the world. The National Institutes of Health (NIH) is the largest single funder of American federal biomedical research, but even within NIH—which is composed of 27 different institutes and centers—project and priority redundancy and fragmentation are likely, as every institute and center receives its own funding and sets its own agenda. This fragmentation may lead to minimal strategy and coordination, increased redundancy, and prioritization of disease areas that are profitable rather than impactful. Strategic coordination across all aspects of the U.S. biomedical research enterprise is necessary to ensure that it is living up to its full potential. Furthermore, this Special Publication argues that dedicated federal funding can significantly impact how Americans are affected—or not—by a specific disease, so the issue of coordination and strategy is not only one of efficiency but also one that may determine the future health and wealth of the nation.

Many of America's peer nations steer their funding and focus with the help of a national-level advisory body and subsequent national strategic vision. The United States currently has neither. Strategic planning at a national scale would enable the United States to be proactive against future health threats, create a communal direction toward achievable goals, improve operational efficiencies, increase productivity, and potentially advance cost-effective health care delivery.

Specifically, a national strategic vision and associated advisory body is necessary to address the increasingly complex health challenges facing Americans, including but not limited to:

- Decreasing life expectancy,
- Women's health issues,
- Persistent health disparities,
- Deaths of despair,
- Obesity,
- Diseases of aging,
- Emerging diseases with pandemic potential, and
- Climate change.

A national strategic vision and advisory body would also enable the direct inclusion of members of the public in discussions about and priority setting for research. Providing opportunities for public input into priorities and execution can ensure that research is relevant to the American people's needs and will help build trust and reassure individuals who are willing to engage directly with the U.S. biomedical research enterprise.

Given the urgency of the health threats facing Americans and the reality of current fragmentation across the biomedical research enterprise, the authors of this Special Publication propose the following:

Priority 1-1: A U.S. biomedical research enterprise advisory body, created by the President of the United States and Congress, to galvanize national leadership, develop a national strategic vision, and coordinate efforts and resources.

Priority 1-2: This advisory body could:
- Be composed of leading scientists from a wide variety of disciplines, such as life, physical, social, and behavioral sciences; engineering; economics; and the humanities to ensure a convergence science approach to addressing all emerging needs;
- Engage with multiple relevant federal agencies;
- Be established with long terms;
- Be empowered to set national goals and benchmarks;
- Provide input on resource allocation that matches strategy;
- Consider, examine, and utilize global best practices in all aspects of its work, but especially as guidance for developing the national strategic vision;
- Include patients, caregivers, and members of the public to provide transparency and public engagement;
- Have clear, measurable goals and timelines;
- Coordinate with the National Economic Policy Council and the Domestic Policy Council to ensure the engagement of all relevant stakeholders; and
- Monitor their progress and report to Congress and the American public annually on their work.

Priority 1-3: The advisory body's national strategic vision could:
- Directly address the current fragmentation in funding and agenda-setting present in the U.S. biomedical research enterprise, in concert with the efforts proposed in Priorities 4-1 and 4-2. The national strategic vision cannot succeed without coordination and alignment of funding and agenda-setting, which, conversely, cannot be coordinated and aligned without the guidance of a national strategic vision. These priorities cannot be separated.
- Set priorities for the use of convergence science and implement a roadmap for bringing together relevant agencies and scientific disciplines to achieve this collaborative approach (see also Priority 4-2).
- Consider and propose funding to address:
  - Existing and emerging health challenges, including but not limited to infant and maternal mortality, women's health concerns, deaths of despair, obesity, climate change, health disparities, diseases with pandemic potential, and diseases of aging;

- Future health threats such as increasing risks of extreme heat and other natural disasters due to climate change and emerging or existing infectious diseases;
- Public engagement in the entire U.S. biomedical research enterprise, but especially focused on increased participation in clinical trials;
- Deteriorating public trust in science and medicine;
- Prioritization and development of new and innovative research approaches to reduce and eliminate health disparities; and
- The needs of the U.S. biomedical research enterprise workforce, including adjusting historical pathways to employment or tenure as emerging health challenges, approaches to science, or the needs of the American public change.

Streamlined and Coordinated Funding

The United States currently spends the most of any country on research and development, but peer nations are increasingly dedicating a higher percentage of their GDP to funding biomedical research. Funding is not everything, but it does enable research to proceed in a focused, stable, and uninterrupted manner. A more streamlined approach to funding research and development, guided by a national body, will help ensure that the U.S. biomedical research enterprise can reach its full potential.

A variety of funding streams flow into U.S. biomedical research, including federal, industry, venture capital, and philanthropy—none of which arrives with "no strings attached." Industry and venture capital funders are driven primarily by returns on investments required by their shareholders. Therefore, they will not or cannot fund a significant portion of biomedical research—particularly early-stage, curiosity-driven discovery research that is critical for advancing science but may have a high likelihood of failure or lack the potential for immediate profits. Alternatively, philanthropy often comes with personal directives that may be limited in scope. This piecemeal funding, driven by a variety of often conflicting agendas, makes it difficult to cobble together sufficient capital to comprehensively address the issues that are most directly impacting Americans.

Relatedly, funding for translating promising basic science into actionable therapeutics, drugs, or diagnostics is often extremely difficult to secure—leading to the funding "valley of death." Many promising breakthroughs often languish between discovery and translation until their promise is recognized—which could be years or decades, if at all. The funding valley of death results in significant waste, because funding and person-power were used to make the discovery, but the discovery is not translated into better health for Americans—or is significantly delayed. Addressing the funding valley of death is critical to ensuring the continuous improvement of the nation's health and will add significant value to what the U.S. biomedical research enterprise is already producing.

To ensure that funding supports the health issues that affect the most Americans and is used to bridge the funding valley of death, the authors of this Special Publication propose the following:

Priority 2-1: A federally established national biomedical research funding collaborative, guided by best practices from existing international models, and federal determinations of how best to organize and allocate shared investments from the government, private sector, and philanthropy. The funding collaborative could be empowered to:
- Analyze successful existing models to develop best practices for the implementation of new methods for financing and accelerating biomedical research;
- Create a large-scale funding model to address the health challenges identified in the national strategic vision; and
- Develop new philanthropic collectives to encourage pooled, strategic gifts that can make a large impact.

Priority 2-2: Federally developed initiatives and funding strategies to specifically address the issue of the "funding valley of death" to translate promising basic research into breakthrough therapies, diagnostics, and treatments—helping to ensure that the full value of the U.S. biomedical research enterprise reaches all patients equitably.

Focus on Health Equity

The successes of the U.S. biomedical research enterprise have not reached all Americans. In fact, some are experiencing increasingly severe health disparities even while others are enjoying improved health. It is time for the U.S. biomedical research enterprise to realize its goal of improving health for *all* Americans and center health equity in its work.

Racial and ethnic minority groups in the United States experience worse outcomes in almost every measure of health and wellness compared to their White counterparts, and women or individuals who identify as women also experience disproportionate health disparities compared to men or individuals who identify as men. These disparities are due to a complex web of factors and are difficult to untangle, understand, and treat. Research focused on reducing health disparities is necessary to better understand how to design and test interventions that can reduce morbidity and mortality for all Americans.

The workforce of the U.S. biomedical research enterprise is also in need of attention as it remains majority White and male. Increasing the diversity of the workforce is not only morally right but also will likely improve outcomes for patients and ensure that research focused on ameliorating health disparities is conducted comprehensively and respectfully. Just as public input is necessary to ensure the success of the national strategic vision, researchers who deeply understand how health and health care are prioritized, viewed, and addressed in their own communities should be involved in developing successful interventions and therapeutics.

The U.S. biomedical research enterprise itself also needs to be examined for issues of equity—specifically regarding the data it collects, aggregates, and uses for research. These data, which are increasingly used to train artificial intelligence models and tools, are not diverse, not representative, and may be race insensitive. Data used throughout the enterprise must represent the actual American populace to advance health equity, reduce health disparities, and design interventions that can successfully address the issues of all Americans.

Lastly, the U.S. biomedical research enterprise must invest in understanding and closing "the last mile"—a critical issue that the authors of this Special Publication have dubbed the "health equity valley of death." Closing the last mile is of equal importance to addressing the funding valley of death because it prevents America's most vulnerable populations from accessing care and the fruits of the U.S. biomedical research enterprise itself. Until the U.S. biomedical research enterprise can address all Americans' unique needs and ensure that the research and products it advances are accessible, it will not have achieved its goal of improving health for all.

To center health equity in all operations of the U.S. biomedical research enterprise and make strides to close the health equity valley of death, the authors of this Special Publication propose the following:

Priority 3-1: Federal prioritization of research that informs solutions for achieving health equity in the United States, including those focused on the social determinants of health, diversifying the workforce, and the U.S. biomedical research enterprise itself. These research areas could include:
- Increasing trust in medicine, science, and the U.S. biomedical research enterprise itself;

- Mitigating structural and systemic discrimination;
- Delivering care to patients and the communities where they reside, using advances in implementation science to guide these solutions;
- Improving the communication of scientific and medical information; and
- Bolstering community engagement and effective bidirectional dialogue.

Priority 3-2: Federal prioritization of research on the "health equity valley of death"—closing the last mile—to understand and eliminate barriers that are preventing the most vulnerable populations in the United States from receiving and accessing comprehensive, high-quality, culturally appropriate care. Specific research areas could include:
- The digital divide;
- Improving access to health care, specifically for individuals who cannot afford adequate or any insurance coverage;
- Transportation barriers;
- "Health care deserts," or a lack of health care providers—primary and specialty—in a given geographic area;
- Improving trust in science, medicine, and practitioners of both;
- Providing care outside of clinics and hospitals to meet individuals where they are; and
- Reducing racism, sexism, and other discriminatory practices that may keep individuals from seeking care.

Improved Federal Coordination and Use of Convergence Science

Suggesting that the federal government needs to coordinate better is an often-recommended improvement; however, for advancing the U.S. biomedical research enterprise, it is a bedrock action. Improved federal coordination is critically necessary for the operation and success of the advisory body and national strategic vision proposed in Priorities 1-1, 1-2, and 1-3 as well as the success of the funding collaborative proposed in Priority 2-1. Implementing these priorities will also ensure more effective and cohesive functioning of all aspects of the U.S. biomedical research enterprise.

Improved federal coordination will also enable the deployment of convergence science to solve the pernicious health challenges currently facing the American public. A National Research Council report defined convergence science as "an approach to problem-solving that integrates expertise from life sciences with physical, mathematical, and computational sciences, medicine, and engineering" as well as social, behavioral, and economic sciences "to form comprehensive synthetic frameworks that merge areas of knowledge from multiple fields to address specific challenges" (NRC, 2014). The report specifically notes that "[a]n enhanced and expanded partnership among convergence practitioners … in the life, physical, and engineering sciences, the economic, social, and behavioral science and humanities research communities, and institutional leaders could be invaluable" (NRC, 2014). The authors of this Special Publication agree. Siloed funding and research agendas, by their nature, prohibit collaboration across federal agencies and areas of expertise—both of which are necessary to solve increasingly complex health issues such as obesity, deaths of despair, and the health impacts of climate change.

Federal coordination and advancement of convergence science will also facilitate the use of public–private partnerships, which provide tremendous opportunities to accelerate discovery and development. Public–private partnerships were implemented during the COVID-19 pandemic, often to great success, but should not be relegated to times of crisis. They should be thoughtfully deployed to address emerging and chronic diseases as well.

To encourage federal coordination and deploy convergence science across all areas of need, the authors of this Special Publication propose the following:

Priority 4-1: Federal requirement and facilitation of necessary and essential coordination across government agencies, especially the National Institutes of Health and the National Science Foundation, as well as external parties, to enable the use of convergence science, coordinate funding and strategy, adequately address the increasingly complex and interconnected health challenges facing the nation, and promote information sharing.

Priority 4-2: Federal promotion and use of convergence science in all appropriate projects receiving federal funding.

21st-Century Workforce

To ensure that the U.S. biomedical research enterprise can continue to produce effective therapeutics, drugs, and diagnostics, it must attract the smartest and most dedicated scientists, researchers, and support staff. However, growth in the biomedical workforce has slowed compared to America's peer nations. Structural compensation, education, and training issues have reached a tipping point and must be addressed before the United States loses competitive applicants to other fields or nations.

International students, scientists, and scholars have contributed significantly to the U.S. biomedical research enterprise. In 2019, more than 4,000 individuals holding temporary visas in the United States were awarded bachelor's degrees in biological sciences; more than 2,500 were awarded master's degrees; and almost 2,000 were awarded doctoral degrees (Trapani and Hale, 2022). Many of these graduates remain in the country for the rest of their professional careers. The biomedical research enterprise must ensure that the United States remains a welcoming and accessible country for international scholars to live, learn, and work.

Fragmented and flat funding for biomedical research also directly impacts the workforce and may influence scientists who are considering careers in biomedical research. The static availability of federal funding may lead to a more cautious approach toward awards, likely harming early-career scientists the most. A coordinated and strategic approach to funding would enable prospective members of the workforce to clearly understand where priorities lie and tailor their research and proposals, if possible.

Lastly, compensation and benefits for entering biomedical research must be raised to parity with similar positions, or the United States will risk losing qualified applicants to industry or academia. Postdoctoral positions regularly pay $15,000 less than comparative positions. Postdoctoral positions—depending on the source of funding—can also vary in access to standard benefits. While most offer health insurance, other benefits such as disability, retirement, or paid leave are not as common. The math here is simple—pay and benefits for these positions must be equivalent to their peer positions, or qualified individuals will move to where the money is.

To ensure a competitive, committed, and well-compensated U.S. biomedical research workforce, the authors of this Special Publication propose the following:

Priority 5: Steps by the federal government and Congress to increase the competitiveness of the U.S. biomedical research enterprise workforce, including the following key priorities:
- Align the U.S. biomedical research enterprise's national strategic vision with the needs of its workforce and set goals to meet those needs;
- Incentivize and implement appropriate, specialized, and necessary education and training for all levels of the U.S. biomedical research workforce—including a reinvigorated focus on K–12 science, technology, engineering, and mathematics education to reinforce the pipeline at its earliest stages;

- Remove barriers that may prevent full accommodation and integration of international scientists into the U.S. biomedical research enterprise workforce, including expanding eligibility for federal research funding to temporary visa holders;
- Expand Early-Stage Investigator funding opportunities, particularly for physician-scientists, to help stabilize the career-launch phase of becoming an independent investigator;
- Reclassify federally funded postdoctoral scholars as employees and provide full benefits to remove unpredictability and make these positions more attractive, including the following potential approaches:
  o Significantly shortening the duration of postdoctoral training so that scholars gain independence faster,
  o Allowing postdoctoral scholars to apply for their own federal funding, and
  o Creating PhD-to-faculty positions, which would provide new pathways to stable employment;
- Promote the importance of physician-scientists to the biomedical research enterprise and support their training, education, and professional work, including the following potential approaches:
  o Expanding and increasing scholarships specifically for physician-scientists,
  o Protecting research time and salary support,
  o Connecting postdoctoral scholars with mentors, and
  o Employing innovative and immersive training and research programs; and
- Prioritize and implement innovative approaches to recruiting and retaining the specialized workforce, including by expanding student loan forgiveness, providing new funding modalities for postdoctoral trainees, and creating early career development awards for new investigators seeking to pursue research fields prioritized by the national strategic vision.

The authors of this Special Publication believe in the strength, power, and impact of the U.S. biomedical research enterprise to support the economy and improve health for all. The actions laid out in this Special Publication, when taken together, will provide the foundation for the U.S. biomedical research enterprise of the future. As a nation, we have already contributed so much—financially, professionally, and personally—to support and advance the enterprise. We owe it to ourselves—and our children and grandchildren—to ensure that biomedical research, conducted effectively, efficiently, and strategically, is benefiting all of America.

1
INTRODUCTION

The U.S. biomedical research enterprise—defined for this Special Publication as individuals and organizations that conduct basic research, applied research, and experimental development as well as the pharmaceutical industry, health care, and public health (see Box 1-1)—contributes to the health of the nation, advances in biomedical and health sciences, and the U.S. economy.

The U.S. biomedical research enterprise has historically been a global leader, and its impacts are far reaching. Beyond health, biomedical research discoveries contribute to advances in agriculture, energy production, and environmental remediation, among other areas. Biomedical research is also an economic engine—generating jobs, innovations, and new technologies—and provides expertise to support governmental priorities during public health crises. Since its inception more than 80 years ago, the U.S. biomedical research enterprise has delivered on its promise to improve human health and has contributed greatly to America's knowledge capital.

However, due to emerging and escalating health crises, global growth in biomedical research that may reduce America's leadership in the field, and existing structural issues that threaten the enterprise's effectiveness and efficiency, attention on how to bolster and streamline the enterprise is needed, which is the focus of this Special Publication.

THE IMPACT OF THE U.S. BIOMEDICAL RESEARCH ENTERPRISE

One way to determine how well the U.S. biomedical research enterprise is performing in terms of improving human health is to identify the top causes of mortality in the United States, the disease areas and National Institutes of Health (NIH) institutes with the highest appropriation levels, and disease prevalence and

> **BOX 1-1**
>
> *Definitions of Types of Research Included in the*
> *U.S. Biomedical Research Enterprise*
>
> - Basic research is "experimental or theoretical work undertaken primarily to acquire new knowledge of the underlying foundations of the phenomena and observable facts, without any particular application or use in view."
> - Applied research is "original investigation undertaken in order to acquire new knowledge. It is, however, directed primarily towards a specific, practical aim or objective."
> - Experimental development is "systematic work, drawing on knowledge gained from research and practical experience and producing additional knowledge, which is directed to producing new products or processes or to improving existing products or processes."
>
> SOURCE: NSF, 2018.

mortality over time. The top two causes of death in the United States in 2019 and 2020 were heart disease and cancer, respectively (see Figure 1-1). HIV/AIDS, although not a current leading cause of death, is a disease that the United States has worked to ameliorate for decades.

Relatedly, three of the consistently highest-funded NIH institutes and centers are the National Cancer Institute (NCI); the National Institute of Allergy and Infectious Diseases (NIAID); and the National Heart, Lung, and Blood Institute (NHLBI) (see Figure 1-2).

The authors of this Special Publication reviewed sufficient data to conclude that significant amounts of sustained federal funding focused on a specific disease or disease type—the primary vehicle by which the U.S. biomedical enterprise funds discovery research—have led to reductions in morbidity and mortality in that disease or disease type. Accordingly, after decades of federal investment in research, education, and prevention, cancer, cardiovascular disease, and HIV/AIDS are no longer death sentences and can be managed as chronic conditions—testaments to the success of the U.S. biomedical research enterprise.

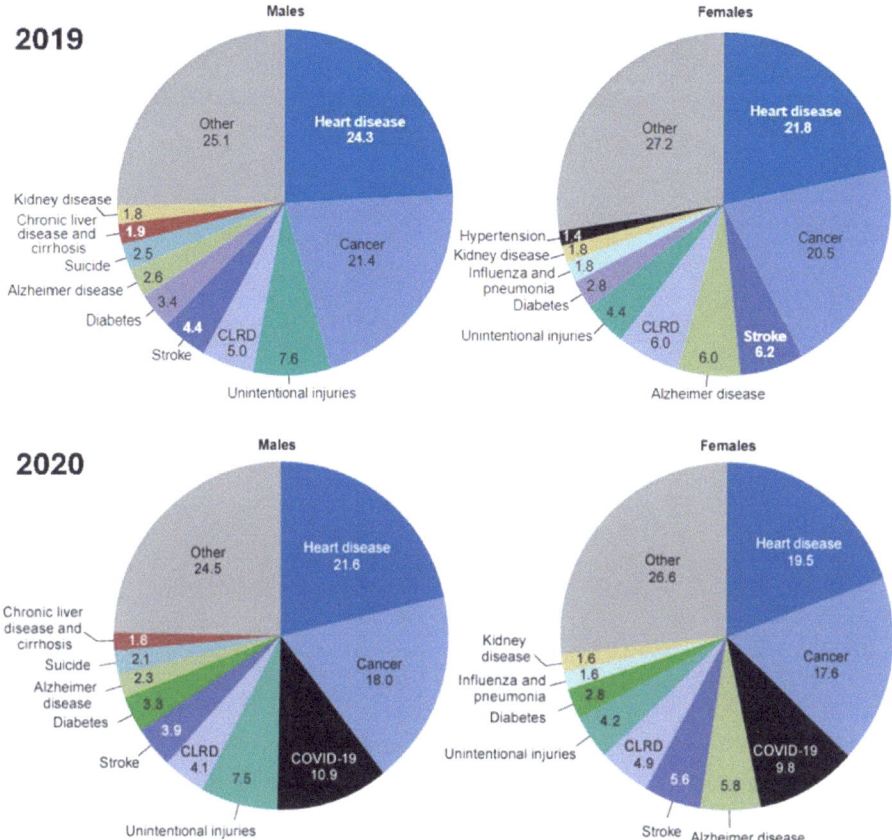

FIGURE 1-1 | Top 10 leading causes of death in the United States, by sex, 2019 and 2020.
NOTES: CLRD = chronic lower respiratory disease. Values show percentage of total deaths.
SOURCES: Curtin et al., 2023; Heron, 2021.

Cancer

Overall, cancer deaths and new cancer cases in the United States have declined in the past two decades (see Figure 1-3). Cancer deaths have declined by 33% since 1991, leading to an estimated 3.8 million more cancer survivors (American Cancer Society, 2023). Many cancers can now be treated without surgery and some—including breast, melanoma, prostate, testicular, and thyroid—have 5-year survival rates above 90% (Kandola, 2023). The 5-year survival rate for all cancers was 49% in the mid-1970s and rose to 68% in 2023 (City of Hope, 2023).

Focused federal attention on addressing cancers began with the 1971 National Cancer Act—legislation that represented America's commitment to the "war

16

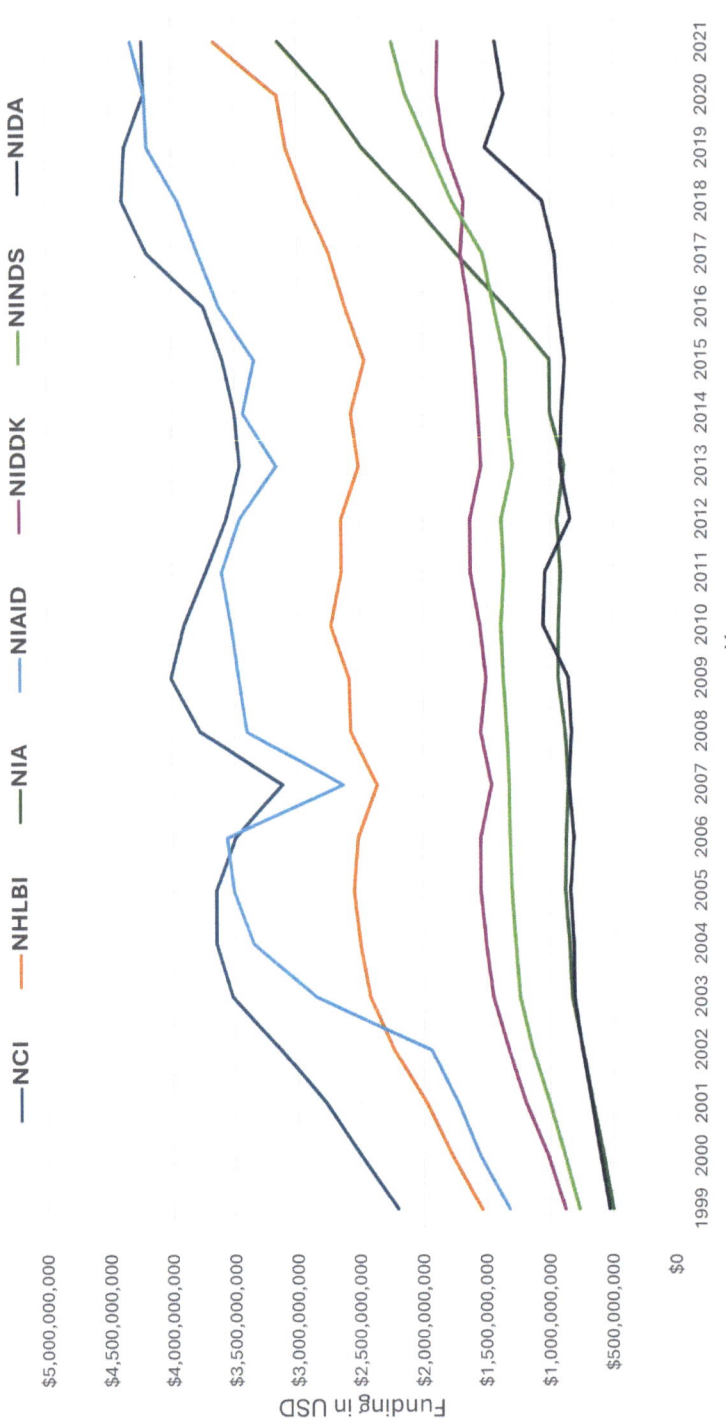

FIGURE 1-2 | National Institutes of Health funding by institute, 1999–2021.
NOTE: NCI = National Cancer Institute; NHLBI = National Heart, Lung, and Blood Institute; NIA = National Institute on Aging; NIAID = National Institute of Allergy and Infectious Diseases; NIDA = National Institute on Drug Abuse; NIDDK = National Institute of Diabetes and Digestive and Kidney Diseases; NINDS = National Institute of Neurological Disorders and Stroke.
SOURCE: NIH, n.d.b.

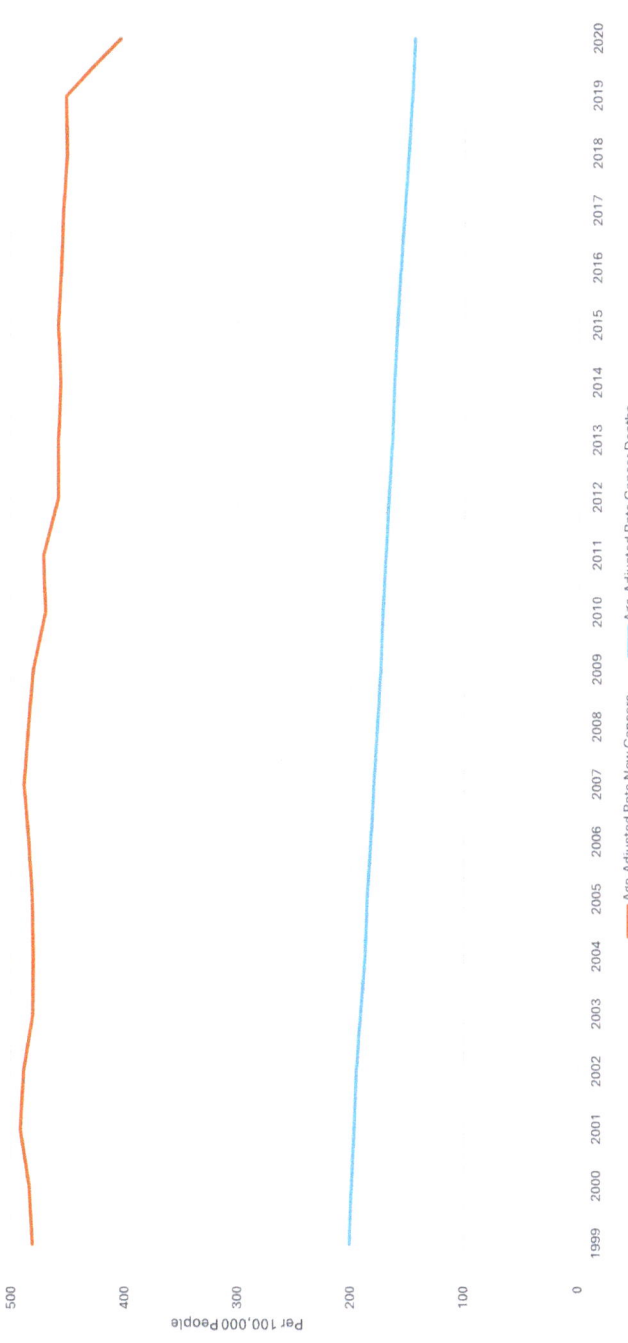

FIGURE 1-3 | Cancer incidence and mortality in the United States, 1999–2021.
NOTE: The orange line represents the number of new cancer cases per 100,000 individuals and the blue line represents the number of cancer deaths per 100,000 individuals.
SOURCE: CDC, 2024d.

on cancer" and allowed for strategic planning; increased funding; and additional researchers, centers, training programs, contracts, and advisory committees to support the increased scope of cancer research (NIH NCI, 2021). The National Cancer Act led to the creation of the NCI Cancer Centers Program, which recognizes high-performing centers utilizing transdisciplinary research (NIH NCI, 2024). Today, 72 NCI-designated cancer centers around the country receive federal funding to perform cancer research and conduct clinical trials to test new cancer treatments (NIH NCI, 2024). In addition to advancing prevention, diagnosis, and treatment, these NCI-funded centers also train the next generation of researchers and clinicians. Collectively, federal funding through NCI that supports education, early screening, research, prevention, and treatment has demonstrably reduced cancer mortality and cancer incidence in the United States.

Cardiovascular Disease

Cardiovascular disease includes coronary heart disease, stroke, high blood pressure, and heart failure, among other conditions (IOM, 2011). Heart disease mortality year over year per 100,000 fell 56% from 307.4 in 1950 to 134.6 in 1996, and stroke rates fell 70% in this same period (Mensah et al., 2017).

Many significant biomedical advances have led to the prevention and treatment of cardiovascular disease, including (examples from Mensah et al., 2017):

- The Framingham Heart Study (1948–current), which identified high blood pressure, high cholesterol, and male gender as major risk factors for cardiovascular disease (NIH NHLBI, n.d.);
- The first coronary artery bypass surgery, performed in 1960 (Konstantinov, 2000); and
- U.S. Food and Drug Administration (FDA) approval of statins in 1987—angiotensin-converting enzyme inhibitors and calcium channel blockers—which are effective drugs for controlling cholesterol and blood pressure and can reduce the incidence of acute cardiovascular disease (Junod, 2007).

NHLBI was created in 1948, after legislation signed by then-President Truman in response to a dramatic increase in American deaths due to cardiovascular disease (NIH NHLBI, 2011). The Framingham Heart Study, in particular, continues to produce valuable data informing current research, as the longitudinal study is now examining the third generation of participants—over 15,000 individuals in total (NIH NHLBI, n.d.). Since its inception, NHLBI has been one of the highest-funded NIH institutes, and this funding has been used to support research that has directly led to the significant reductions in morbidity and mortality described above (NIH OB, n.d.).

HIV/AIDS

HIV/AIDS has claimed 700,000 U.S. lives since the beginning of the epidemic in 1981, but HIV infection can now be largely prevented and managed as a chronic condition (KFF, 2021). In 2019, the death rate due to HIV/AIDS was 1.4 per 100,000—a reduction from the highest point of 16.2 per 100,000 in 1995 (Walker, n.d.). In addition to significantly reducing the death rate due to HIV/AIDS infection, 50 drugs are now available for managing HIV levels—compared to just 1 in 1987 (FDA, 2019; HIVinfo.NIH.gov, 2023).

There were few effective therapies for AIDS in the late 1980s, but the Health Omnibus Programs Extension was passed in 1988 and extended in 1993, establishing the Office of AIDS Research at NIH and leading to a strategic plan, budget, and coordinated research around HIV and AIDS (NIH OAR, 2023). Due to the focused effort of the Office of AIDS Research, significant federal funding, and the participation of many other NIH institutes, protease inhibitors were discovered in 1996, which extend the lives of people living with HIV/AIDS (NIH, 2015). Researchers at NIAID also contributed to developing a wide variety of antiviral drugs, as "HIV mutates rapidly and some people can't tolerate certain drugs," so "cocktails" of medications are necessary to treat people living with HIV/AIDS (Collins and Fauci, 2010). More recently, better access to HIV testing, increased access to treatment, improved education about HIV/AIDS, and the use of pre-exposure prophylaxis—or PrEP—have led to further declines in infection rates (Park, 2023).

Basic Science and Future Discoveries

The steady advance of biomedical research has also enabled many critical discoveries that would have been impossible without decades of quiet and unpublicized research and funding. Most notably, years of basic science underpinned the unprecedented rapidity in developing safe and effective vaccinations against COVID-19. The fundamental research in mRNA technology that served as the basis for the platforms that ultimately produced effective vaccines was performed before 2000 (WHO, 2023a). These types of discoveries—often unheralded by the public—coupled with effective public–private partnerships resulted in millions of lives saved globally (No author, 2022a). This is just one example that illustrates the continued promise of the U.S. biomedical research enterprise in reducing mortality, if appropriately funded and coordinated.

HISTORY AND CURRENT STATE OF THE U.S. BIOMEDICAL RESEARCH ENTERPRISE

The path to the U.S. biomedical research enterprise that achieved the successes outlined above has been winding. The structure of the enterprise was established in the 1940s under President Roosevelt's direction with the creation of the Office of Scientific Research and Development (OSRD) to leverage and coordinate scientific research for military purposes. The work of the OSRD led to scientific advances such as the creation of radar and the mass manufacturing of penicillin to treat infectious diseases (Hourihan, 2020). On the heels of the Second World War, President Roosevelt asked Vannevar Bush—a mathematician, electrical engineer, and then-director of OSRD—to propose how the United States could leverage the wartime research and development (R&D) effort during peacetime. Bush's report, *Science: The Endless Frontier*, outlined a central role for the government in developing scientific talent, funding basic research in institutions of higher education, and supporting new scholarships and fellowships to ensure that talent would not be prevented from entering the field by financial hardship (Bush, 1945). Bush's recommendations led to the creation of the National Science Foundation (NSF)—an organization dedicated to funding basic research (NSF, n.d.). Bush's bold blueprint for American scientific research laid the foundation for decades of innovation and U.S. leadership in science, technology, and health care.

In parallel, a growing "citizen science" movement led by advocates and philanthropists such as Mary Lasker and Florence Mahoney helped promote government-sponsored medical research and the creation of NIH (Harman and Dietrich, 2018). At the time, many scientists opposed government involvement in research. Lasker, however, famously argued, "if you think research is expensive, try disease," in lobbying for the U.S. government to play a central role in supporting research to proactively shoulder some of the cost burdens of illness (Haley, 2022). In response to these efforts, the 1944 Public Health Service Act consolidated previously disparate efforts in medical research under the single administrative structure of the National Institute of Health (the predecessor to the National Institutes of Health)—including the previously established National Cancer Institute (NIH, 2024a). Beginning in 1946, Lasker and Mahoney pivoted to lobbying for NIH to expand to include multiple institutes focusing on different aspects of health, resulting in the Omnibus Medical Research Act in 1950, which established the National Institute of Neurological Diseases and Blindness and the National Institute of Arthritis and Metabolic Diseases and opened the door for the creation of other institutes, including the National Institute of Allergy and Infectious Diseases in 1955 (NIH, 2024a). The National Heart Institute was established separately in 1948 (NIH, 2024a). Between 1945 and 1961 NIH congressional appropriations increased 150-fold to $450 million, reaching approximately $1 billion by the late 1960s (NIH OB, n.d.). By 1960, the United States accounted for approximately 69% of all global scientific R&D, and the rest of the globe combined contributed the remaining 31% (CRS, 2022). See Figure 1-4 for a visual trend of NIH funding between 1938 and 1961.

In 2005, in response to growing concerns about declining U.S. investment in research and higher education and the competitiveness of U.S. businesses within the global market, the Senate Committee on Energy and Natural Resources and the House Committee on Science asked the National Academies of Sciences, Engineering, and Medicine to identify and prioritize 10 top actions that could enhance the science and technology enterprise. The resulting consensus study, *Rising Above the Gathering Storm: Energizing and Employing America for a Brighter Future*, was published in 2007 and updated in 2010 (NAS et al., 2007, 2010). The committee asserted that "innovation, largely derived from advances in science and engineering," is a primary driver of the U.S. economy (NAS et al., 2010). However, the 2007 report also noted two potentially troubling facts—that federal sources funded 60% of U.S. R&D in 1965 but dropped below 30% by 2002, and that in many science and engineering fields, 38% of those receiving PhDs from American universities were foreign scholars (NAS et al., 2007).

The 2007 report informed and helped establish the America COMPETES Act of 2007, which authorized $33.6 billion in appropriations and a 10.4% funding growth rate for a projected 7-year doubling of the NSF and the Department of Energy's Office of Science budgets (CRS, 2015). The Act also authorized, for the first time, the Advanced Research Projects Agency–Energy, which "advances high-potential, high-impact energy technologies that are too early for private-sector investment" (ARPA-E, n.d.). Unfortunately, the Act was not fully funded or implemented (CRS, 2015).

In 2015, Hamilton Moses III and colleagues published a special communication in *JAMA* that called for "new investment … if the clinical value of past scientific discoveries and opportunities to improve care are to be fully realized" (Moses et al., 2015). The authors argued that research conducted by U.S. academic medical centers—often funded by federal monies—remains the cornerstone of innovation and advancement of new therapeutics, devices, and procedures and represents the hallmark of what makes U.S. research distinct from that of other nations.

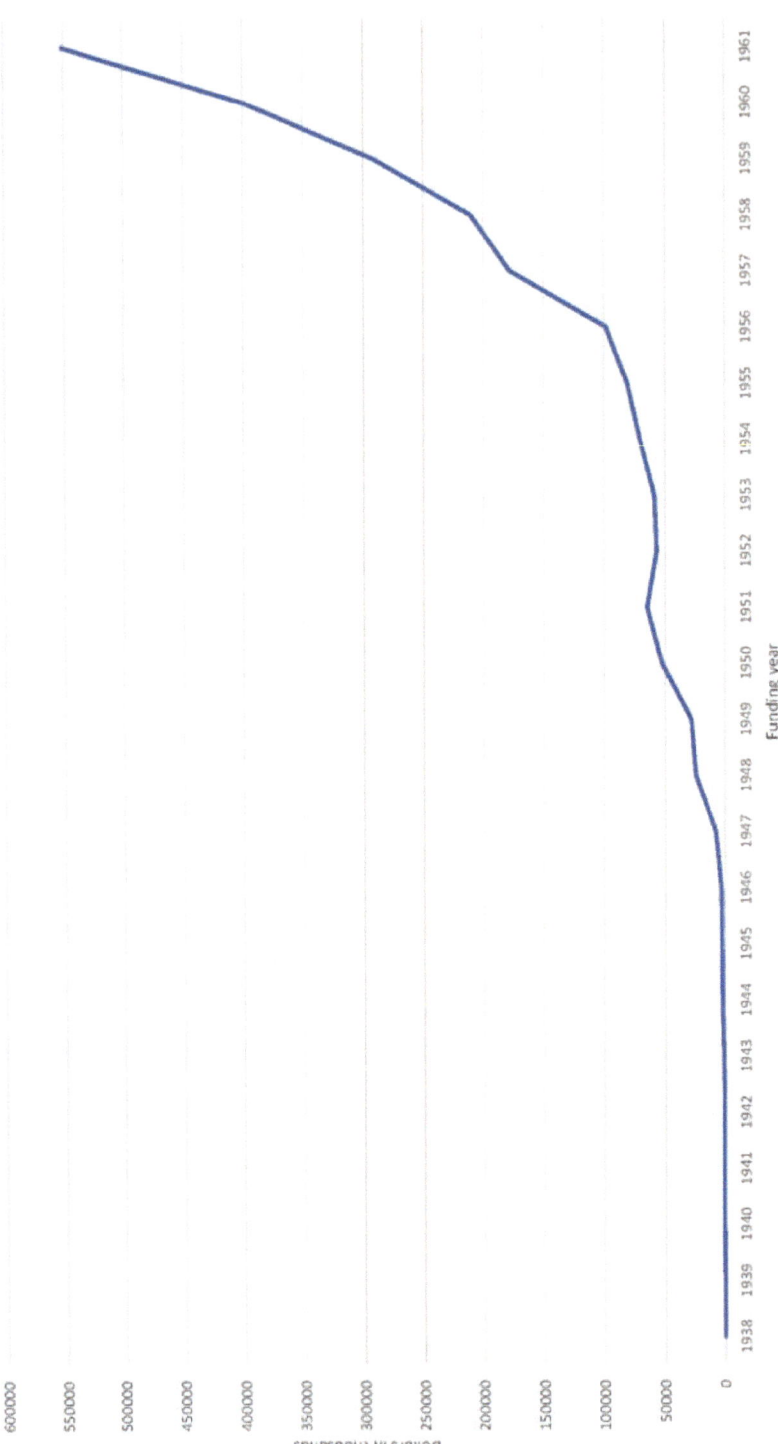

FIGURE 1-4 | National Institutes of Health funding by year.
DATA SOURCE: NIH OB, n.d.

Advent of Precision Medicine:
A Major Milestone in the History of the
U.S. Biomedical Research Enterprise

The Human Genome Project (HGP), improvements in computational biology, and the availability of genomic data have recently enabled researchers to improve their ability to predict the combined effects of many gene variants that make up an individual's genome and calculate the likelihood of developing certain diseases, how severe that disease will be, and how quickly it might progress. These improvements have led to increasingly individualized care for each patient—broadly known as precision medicine—which holds great promise for improving population health.

HGP was an international effort led by the United States to decode the entire human genome, and has, since its inception, continued to change health and medicine (NIH NHGRI, 2024). HGP—launched in 1990, completed in 2003, and funded by the U.S. federal government—provided the first comprehensive map of all the genes in the human genome, which enabled researchers to identify molecular mechanisms underlying disease in individuals, deconstructing the traditional "one-size-fits-all" approach to medicine (NIH NHGRI, 2024). This information will, ideally, lead to a new approach to health care that can provide each patient with a treatment plan tailored to their disease, information on their risks of developing certain diseases, and guidance on what could be done to delay or mitigate disease. While each person's genome holds hereditary information about their risks for certain conditions, the social determinants of health—including where people are born, where they live and work, and other non-medical factors—also contribute to an individual's overall health status (Chelak and Chakole, 2023). All these data will be critical for realizing the promise of individualized approaches to maintaining a person's best health.

Although researchers will continue to translate genomic knowledge into clinical practice for decades to come, many discoveries from HGP have already had far-reaching impacts. These early advances have led to a better understanding of genetics, genomics, and disease; the development of new diagnostic and therapeutic strategies; and new models for data sharing. The following list describes some paradigm-shifting early advances:

- Polygenic risk scores—a predictive likelihood of developing certain diseases—have been calculated for hypothyroidism, hypertension, type 1 and 2 diabetes, breast cancer, prostate cancer, testicular cancer, gallstones, glaucoma, gout, atrial fibrillation, high cholesterol, asthma, basal cell carcinoma, malignant melanoma, and heart attack (Lello et al., 2019). These scores can inform treatment decisions by identifying people with high genetic risks of developing disease—enabling earlier intervention—and identifying individuals who may not respond to certain drugs and will require differential treatments (Lello et al., 2019).

- Much like the tests for identifying BRCA1 and BRCA2—genetic variants that signal a higher risk for developing breast cancer—researchers have leveraged genomic information to develop genetic tests for other inherited conditions. In 2012, a total of 607 genetic tests were available in the United States—in 2022, a total of 51,803 genetic tests were available (Halbisen and Lu, 2023).
- Researchers are also using their detailed knowledge of gene sequences—derived from HGP—alongside clustered regularly interspaced short palindromic repeats (CRISPR) gene editing to potentially correct gene defects and ameliorate disease. In September 2023, a clinical trial to treat acute lymphoblastic leukemia with a genetically engineered chimeric antigen receptor T-cell (CAR-T) therapy began, and in May 2024, the first patient in the United States received a gene therapy to hopefully cure sickle cell disease (Beam Therapeutics, 2023; Kolata, 2024).
- Whole tumor sequencing of cancer patients has led to The Cancer Genome Atlas, which helped identify the most commonly mutated genes that appear to accelerate disease (NIH NCI, n.d.a). The Atlas also enables researchers to identify rare mutations. This collection of data has helped identify targets for developing new drugs and highlighted genetic variants that indicate how well certain drugs will work.

THE U.S. BIOMEDICAL RESEARCH ENTERPRISE IS AN ENGINE FOR THE U.S. ECONOMY

When speaking about the "value" of the U.S. biomedical research enterprise, a healthy nation is the most desirable outcome. However, the authors of this Special Publication also believe that financial growth will follow as health improves. Healthier people are more productive, earn more, and live longer (Braveman et al., 2018). The longer people live, the more they earn, and the more they can save and increase capital. The lifetime potential contribution per person in the United States is $1.5 million in productivity (Grosse et al., 2018). Public health studies of low-income countries have shown that a 10% increase in life expectancy at birth corresponds to a 1% increase in annual gross domestic product (GDP) per capita growth in 5 years and 0.4% in additional growth over 35 years (Bloom et al., 2020).

The association between reducing mortality and improved economic impact is not just an American phenomenon. An economic analysis of health and labor productivity in Australia, Denmark, Finland, France, Italy, Japan, the Netherlands, Norway, Sweden, and the United Kingdom found that a 10% increase in adult survival during their working years would lead to a 6.7% increase in productivity per worker and an increase of 4.4% GDP per worker (Weil, 2007).

Closer to home, an analysis of the Blue Cross Blue Shield Health Index also shows a strong relationship between health and economic performance. The Index comprises deidentified annual data from 43 million Blue Cross Blue Shield members—not including those insured by Medicaid and Medicare—their health status related to more than 390 health conditions, and medical and pharmacy claims data (BlueCross BlueShield, 2024). An analysis by Moody's reveals that U.S. counties with the highest health scores—defined by the ratio of "expected remaining healthy years of life divided by the number of years that an individual would have under optimal health"—had average incomes that were nearly $4,000 higher than the national average, and the GDPs of the counties themselves were almost $10,000 higher than the national average (White and Ozimek, 2016). The analysis also found that low unemployment rates are associated with higher health scores (White and Ozimek, 2016). Counties with average health scores in the 99th percentile—with 100% being the highest possible health score and 0% being the lowest—are associated with an increase in average annual pay of $5,302 and a 0.6% decline in unemployment (White and Ozimek, 2016).

The U.S. biomedical research enterprise also contributes directly to the U.S. economy. NIH-funded discoveries comprise much of the foundation of the enterprise, contributing $69 billion to America's GDP and supporting 7 million jobs (NIH, 2023a). NIH-funded discoveries also regularly lead to new drug development, providing a 43% return on public investment, per data spanning from 1980 to 2005 (Azoulay et al., 2019). The $37.81 billion in extramural research support provided by NIH for fiscal year 2023 directly and indirectly supported more than 412,000 jobs nationally, producing new economic activity across all 50 states and the District of Columbia (United for Medical Research, 2024).

The U.S. biomedical and pharmaceutical private sector generated more than $1.4 trillion in economic output in 2020, which brought in $76 billion in tax revenues (PhRMA and Teconomy Partners LLC, 2022). This sector employs more than 903,000 individuals directly and supports, indirectly, an additional 3.5 million jobs (PhRMA and Teconomy Partners LLC, 2022).

Intangible capital—including data, patents, copyrights, and other non-physical capital—has increased over the past several decades and has grown to be increasingly important in valuations of the U.S. biomedical research enterprise. Ståhle and colleagues estimate that intangible capital accounts for 45% of the global GDP and as much as 70% of the U.S. GDP (Ståhle et al., 2015).

There is tremendous value in a healthy population, and this value can be approximated but not truly measured. However, existing data clearly show that investing in individual and population health does improve economic strength. In the United States, strong historical investment in the biomedical research enterprise has improved health and reduced mortality. It follows that strong investments will ensure continued health and economic prosperity.

WHY DOES THE U.S. BIOMEDICAL RESEARCH ENTERPRISE NEED ATTENTION IN 2024?

Despite the successes outlined above, issues have arisen that require the renewed attention of the U.S. biomedical research enterprise—and to the function and structure of the enterprise itself. These issues include increasing competitiveness from other nations in terms of R&D, scientific advances, and funding; emerging and intensifying health threats that require the use of convergence science in brand new ways; and existing and historical structural issues within the enterprise that prevent its utmost effectiveness, including strategy, workforce, health equity, and funding. This Special Publication outlines these issues, why they are so critical, and what actions can be taken in the near and medium terms to address them.

The health challenges facing the United States are no more complex than those we have made progress in treating—the difference is how far biomedical research has advanced. The artificial intelligence and health technology revolution, combined with major advances in fields such as -omics biology and precision medicine, have fundamentally changed how medicine is studied and practiced. To advance in parallel, the U.S. biomedical research enterprise itself needs to grow and change.

VISION FOR THE U.S. BIOMEDICAL RESEARCH ENTERPRISE OF THE FUTURE

The authors of this Special Publication believe that action is needed in the short and medium terms to revitalize, reinvigorate, and shore up the U.S. biomedical research enterprise. If the actions proposed within this Special Publication are taken, the authors believe that the vision of the U.S. biomedical research enterprise presented below is well within reach (see Figure 1-5).

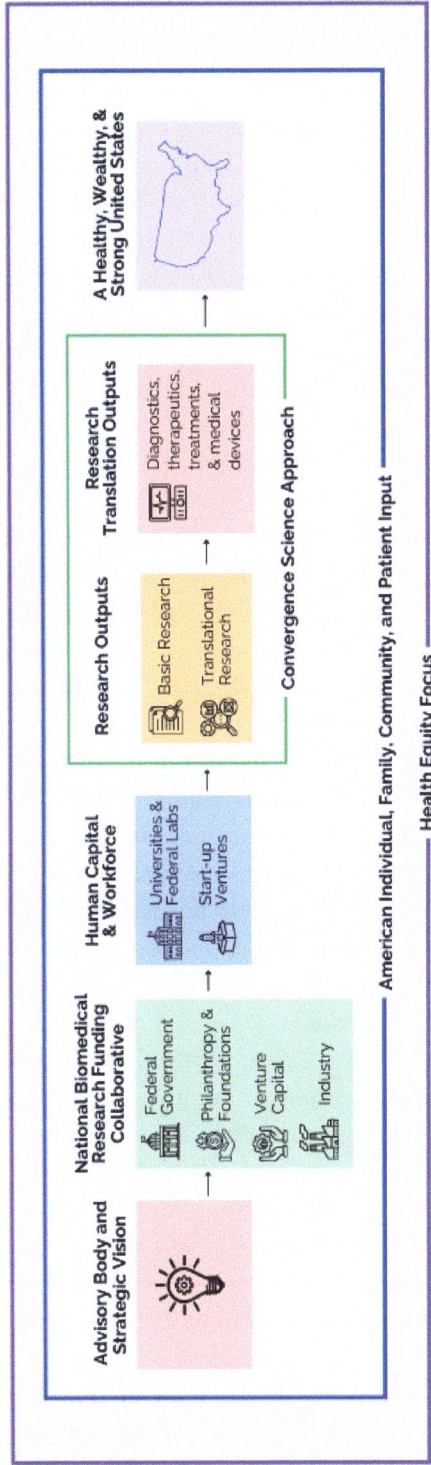

FIGURE 1-5 | Future state of the U.S. biomedical research enterprise.

Vision for the Future

The Pioneer 100 Wellness program, launched by the Institute for Systems Biology, has conclusively shown that leveraging genomic data, emerging technology, and improved understanding of disease mechanisms can improve health—a snapshot of what the future U.S. biomedical research enterprise could be. In 2013, the Institute for Systems Biology team recruited 108 people to have their genomes sequenced and measures of health analyzed for 9 months (Hood and Price, 2023). Participants wore activity trackers to measure their sleep, activity, and heart rate (Hood and Price, 2023). The researchers collected blood, saliva, and stool from each participant to measure and analyze "1,200 blood analytes—proteins, metabolites, and other clinically relevant chemicals," including cortisol and the number and types of bacteria in their gut microbiomes (Hood and Price, 2023). A wellness and nutrition coach used these measurements to develop individual action plans for each participant and "persuade the pioneers to change their lifestyles in accordance with the individual recommendations"—whether they were at risk for diabetes or another disease, or simply lacking specific nutrients (Hood and Price, 2023).

Of the 108 participants, 53 had prediabetes. By the end of the 9-month intervention period, 38% improved their blood glucose levels, 55% improved their insulin resistance, and 7 individuals had reversed the presence of prediabetes entirely (Hood and Price, 2023). The personalized action plans resulted in a 12% improvement in the presence of inflammation biomarkers that are associated with Alzheimer's disease, cancer, heart disease, and diabetes; a 6% improvement for markers associated with coronary artery disease; and a 21% improvement for markers associated with improved nutrition (Hood and Price, 2023).

Imagine if every American could have access to individualized action plans such as these to improve their health.

Imagine if every American had enough trust in the U.S. biomedical research enterprise to contribute their genomic, health, and medical data to advance precision medicine and machine learning. This robust data set could reveal opportunities for everyone to enhance their health and provide the ability to predict, prevent, and precisely mitigate disease development. A future health care delivery system would partner with individuals, enabling them to take control of their health by providing specific plans to prevent or mitigate disease. When disease did occur, health care systems would provide therapies designed to treat their exact condition, precisely.

Imagine a health care delivery system focused on enhancing health and longevity while preventing disease instead of waiting until people are sick to treat them. This approach would not only improve the health of the nation but also potentially save hundreds of billions of dollars and reduce the more than 17% of GDP the United States currently spends on health care (CMS, 2023).

Imagine not only increasing individual life expectancy but also reducing the ill health that typically accompanies aging—including chronic diseases, dementias, frailty, and disability. Unveiling the biology of aging could provide essential knowledge toward delaying aging and its consequences, leading to a better health span for all.

Imagine the 58.5 million Americans who currently live with arthritis, one of the top three causes of work disability, being able to work without pain, saving $164 billion in lost earnings and immeasurably improving their quality of life (Murphy et al., 2018; Theis et al., 2018).

Imagine the 37 million Americans living with diabetes in 2022 earning the $28.3 billion lost because they could not work due to disability, and being able to spend more hours, days, and years with their friends and families (DRIF, 2023; Parker et al., 2023).

Imagine eliminating the health disparities that cause 30% more Black individuals to die from cardiovascular disease than their White peers; American Indian or Alaska Native individuals to develop diabetes at twice the rate of their White peers; and American Indian or Alaska Native, Hispanic, and Black individuals to be more than 1.5 times as likely to die from COVID-19 as their White peers (HHS OMH, n.d.; Hill et al., 2023; Terrie, 2023).

Imagine strategic investments to support improvements in health that will not only save lives and improve quality of life but also bolster individual wealth, eliminate unnecessary costs, and improve the economy. **We can achieve this vision if we act now.**

2
A STRATEGIC AND COORDINATED APPROACH TO THE U.S. BIOMEDICAL RESEARCH ENTERPRISE

To achieve the vision for an improved and more robust U.S. biomedical research enterprise laid out in Chapter 1, the federal government, academia, philanthropy, venture capital, and all other stakeholders must consider and plan for America's needs in a more coordinated, thoughtful, and strategic manner.

FRAGMENTATION STANDS IN THE WAY OF MAXIMUM POTENTIAL

The collective investment of the federal government, venture capital, industry, and philanthropy into the biomedical research enterprise is significant—in 2019, U.S. spending accounted for 27% of the global total investment in research and development (R&D), the highest absolute dollar investment of any country (NSF NSB, 2022).

Despite this massive investment, the "buckets" of money committed to the enterprise in the United States sometimes have competing priorities, diluting the effectiveness of such a remarkable amount of money. The type of funding source—even inadvertently—can influence research priorities, goals, and approaches—for better or worse. Not all agendas benefit all stakeholders, because each sector has its own priorities for spending.

For example, the private sector—including biotechnology, pharmaceuticals, and venture capital—is driven by market pressures and returns on investment, and therefore focuses primarily on research that will result in products, including therapeutics and devices. Although these therapeutics and devices are usually available to all consumers, industry-driven basic research often relates directly to business strategies and is therefore confidential, which contributes in a siloed and skewed manner to the U.S. knowledge capital and may not benefit other researchers.

In contrast, the goal of the National Institutes of Health (NIH)—the largest federal funder of the biomedical research enterprise—is to seek fundamental knowledge and apply that knowledge broadly (NIH, 2017). Interpreted narrowly, that goal might include only basic research, but NIH actually funds everything from basic to applied research. Per NIH's data, the distribution of its budget spent on basic versus applied research over the past 20 years has ranged from approximately 60–40 to approximately 50–50 (Lauer, 2023) (see Figure 2-1). NIH-funded research is publicly available to anyone who is interested in accessing the data and findings, and much—although not all—of the research does not directly result in an immediately marketable product.

Philanthropic gifts, although often given with significantly fewer restrictions than private- or public-sector funds, are often driven by personal desires, experiences, or emotions. For example, gifts may be given by grateful patients to individual researchers rather than an overall institution, or larger gifts may be restricted to focusing only on one disease state or type of disease, disallowing the use of those funds for emerging or urgent issues.

Because the goals and approach of the public, private, and philanthropic sectors in biomedical research are at odds, it is easy to see how fragmentation could occur and how these drivers could lead to outcomes that do not serve the greatest social need. However, the issue is deeper still. Even within the government agency that funds most biomedical research, fragmentation likely abounds. Each of NIH's 27 institutes is responsible for setting much of its research agenda (NIH, 2018). The Division of Program Coordination, Planning, and Strategic Initiatives within NIH exists to help coordinate research around "emerging scientific opportunity or rising public health challenges" but it is easy to imagine duplicative, overlapping, or conflicting research projects being funded by different NIH institutes (NIH, 2018).

The siloed nature of these funding sources, conflicting agendas, and the lack of a cohesive strategy with buy-in from all stakeholders is concerning, because addressing the emerging, complex health conditions plaguing the American people will require sustained, coordinated, and focused research involving scientists from many different backgrounds.

THE ROLE OF NIH

Because NIH, via the Department of Health and Human Services, is the largest federal funder of American biomedical research, its structure and function have been central to setting biomedical research priorities and agendas since its inception (NSF NSB, 2020). As mentioned above, Congress allocates funding

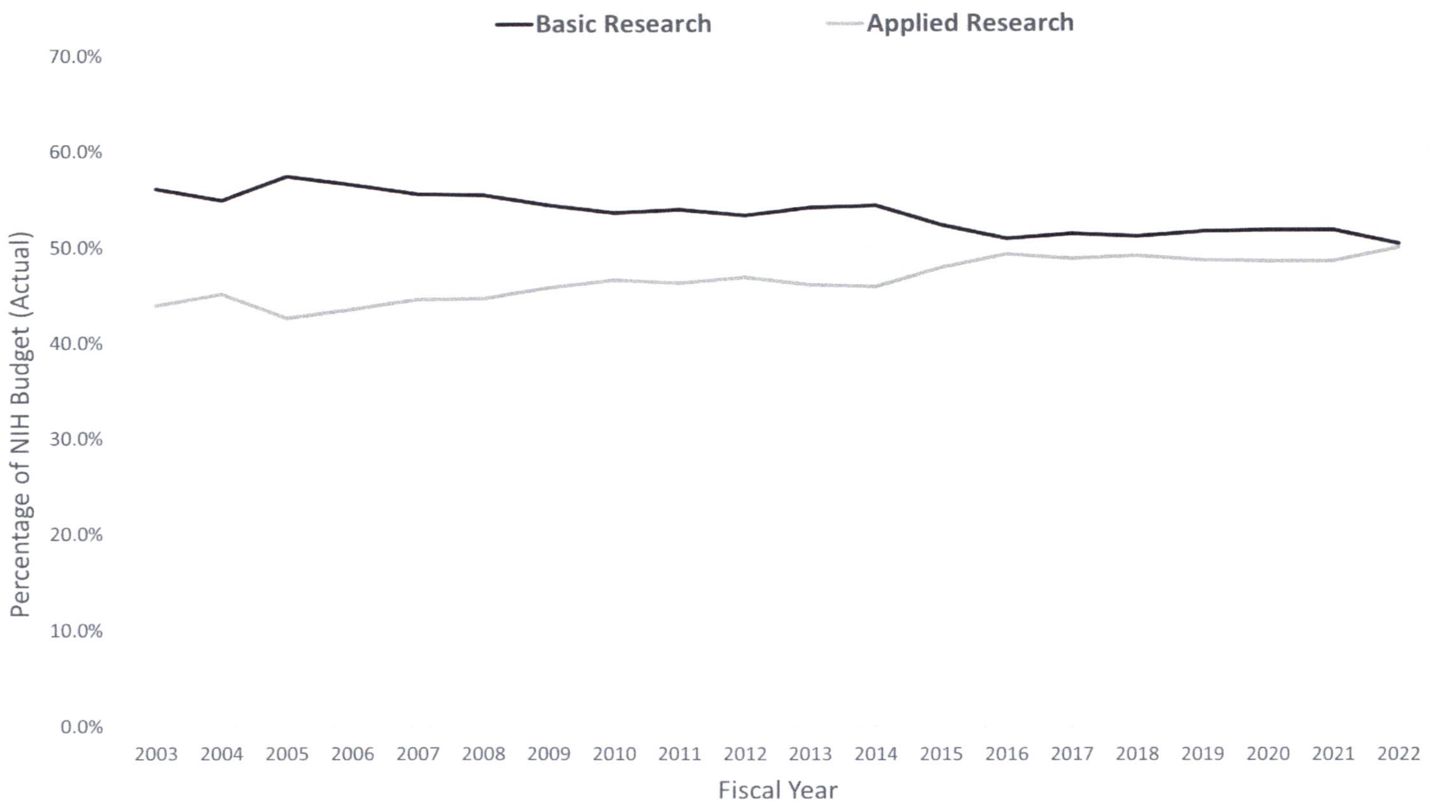

FIGURE 2-1 | National Institutes of Health spending on basic and applied research, 2003–2022.
NOTE: The proportion of the actual NIH budget spent on basic (black line) and applied (gray line) research.
DATA SOURCE: NIH, 2023b.

to individual NIH institutes, which are then empowered to set their research agendas and allocate much of their funding themselves. Some institutes have historically and regularly received larger allocations than other institutes (including the National Cancer Institute [NCI] and the National Heart, Lung, and Blood Institute [NHLBI], outlined in Chapter 1) which have enabled them to grow both in terms of employees and research portfolios, which then require even larger allocations in the future (NIH OB, n.d.). Allocating funding strictly based on the size of the NIH institute may not necessarily serve the greatest public good at the time, because emerging issues may fall under the umbrella of less-well-funded institutes.

The topline NIH budget also includes funding for infrastructure and special projects such as the Cancer Moonshot and pandemic preparedness, which do not require cross-agency coordination—or the Cancer Moonshot and cancer efforts at the Advanced Research Projects Agency for Health that distribute funding across agencies and may fragment what should be cohesive and coordinated efforts (NIH NCI, n.d.b; The White House, 2023). Appropriations bills can add specific text to direct how NIH institutes spend their budgets, and lobbying groups and other nonprofit coalitions go directly to Congress to push disease-specific agendas, which can receive different degrees of attention depending on how disease-specific agendas originate, thus resulting in different degrees of funding success during the appropriations process (Wouters, 2020). These many competing priorities and the lack of a central strategy often lead to complex, layered agenda-setting and may result in appropriations that do not entirely or accurately reflect overarching national needs.

As established in Chapter 1, dedicated federal funding is likely to significantly impact how Americans are impacted by a specific disease. For example, funding for NCI and NHLBI has increased dramatically since 2000, and mortality rates for both cancer and cardiovascular diseases have, overall, declined (CDC, 2024a; NIH NCI, 2023; NIH NHLBI, 2024). Even though the direct correlation between funding and mortality is difficult to calculate, it seems that these long-standing institutes with significant federal budget allocations have contributed to decreased mortality. Lower funding levels and/or lower funding increases are also reflected in disease mortality data, which suggest that deliberate attention and associated appropriations are required to address America's emerging health challenges. For example, since 2000, the age-adjusted prevalence of diabetes has significantly increased among adults aged 18 years and older, but NIDDK has one of the lowest rates of funding increase among the NIH institutes—from $1.693 billion in fiscal year 2013 to $2.3 billion in fiscal year 2023 (NIH NIDDK, 2013, 2024).

Sustained and robust investments in NIH have led to the training of thousands of biomedical- and physician-scientists, effective therapies for diseases that were once death sentences, and, more recently, the rapid development of effective COVID-19 vaccines. A thriving U.S. biomedical research enterprise also created a strong U.S. knowledge capital, robust biotechnology and pharmaceutical industries, and hundreds of thousands of high-wage jobs, and continues to add billions of dollars each year to the U.S. gross domestic product (GDP) (The Science Coalition, 2024). Without clear, overarching goals guided by a thoughtful and coordinated central strategic vision, too many priorities compete for a limited pool of funds. This competition may lead NIH to hedge its bets and award funding to relatively safe and incremental proposals—rather than research that is risky but could advance the biomedical enterprise in bold and rewarding ways. A national strategic vision could also help NIH and other funders better understand which investments would most benefit the American public—even if, or especially if, those investments do not track with the size or longevity of a certain focus area.

WHY A NATIONAL STRATEGIC VISION IS NECESSARY

The United States needs to break down existing funding, information, and coordination silos to support the success of a national strategic vision for the biomedical research enterprise—under which many current efforts can continue. Strategic planning at a national scale would enable the entire biomedical research enterprise to be proactive against future health threats, create a communal direction toward achievable goals, improve operational efficiencies, increase productivity, and advance cost-effective health care delivery. Likewise, national-scale strategic planning could and should be used to determine the amount of biomedical research funding required over time. The current economic and public health climates heighten the urgency for the U.S. government to seize the opportunity to establish a national strategic vision so that impending threats, such as those that follow, can be ameliorated.

American Life Expectancy Is Falling

By most health metrics, the U.S. population faces several significant health challenges—many of which are reflected in life expectancy, which is generally seen as a bellwether for the overall health of a nation. An analysis conducted by *The Washington Post* in 2023 found that American life expectancy has been falling for the past decade compared to other wealthy nations (Achenbach et al., 2023). Life expectancy in 2010 in the United States was 78.6 years, compared to 80.2 in

Germany, 81.3 in Canada, and 82.2 in Switzerland (WHO, 2020). In 2022, life expectancy in the United States was 77.5, down 1.1 from 2010 (Peterson-KFF Health System Tracker, 2024). Comparatively, in 2022 Germany and Switzerland's life expectancy rose to 80.8 and 83.5, respectively, and Canada's life expectancy stayed stable at 81.3 (Peterson-KFF Health System Tracker, 2024).

Life expectancy also differs significantly between racial and ethnic groups. Within the United States, provisional data for 2021 show a decline in U.S. life expectancy since 2019 of 6.6 years for American Indian and Alaska Native individuals, 4.2 years for Hispanic individuals, 4 years for Black individuals, 2.4 years for White individuals, and 2.1 years for Asian individuals (Arias et al., 2022). This continued decline—and associated disparities—requires prompt attention.

Women's Health Concerns Are Growing and Poorly Understood

Although women comprise more than half of the U.S. population, conditions that disproportionately impact women and individuals who identify as women are under-researched and underdiagnosed (Blakeslee et al., 2023; Whiting, 2024). Additionally, although U.S. women experience longer life expectancy than men do, between 2021 and 2022, male life expectancy increased by 1.3 years, compared to only 0.9 years in women (see Figure 2-2). This apparent slowing of life expectancy growth is further complicated by the fact that "women spend 25% more of their lives in debilitating health than men," meaning that despite their longer lives, women generally experience poorer health spans than men do (Whiting, 2024).

According to the National Health Interview Survey conducted annually by the Centers for Disease Control and Prevention, women fare worse than men in many aspects of health, including respiratory diseases, cancer, arthritis, and obesity (see Table 2-1). More women than men also reported that they have only fair or poor health and that they did not receive needed medical care due to cost (see Table 2-1).

Diseases and conditions that exclusively or disproportionately affect female patients and/or patients who identify as women receive significantly less federal funding than diseases exclusively or predominantly affecting male patients and/or patients who identify as men (Smith, 2023; Temkin et al., 2023). Likewise, an analysis of cancer funding showed that gynecological cancers are not as well funded as other cancers when considering their lethality (Rush et al., 2021).

The United States spends more on health care per capita than any other high-income country—"on average, other large, wealthy countries spent about half

A Strategic and Coordinated Approach | 37

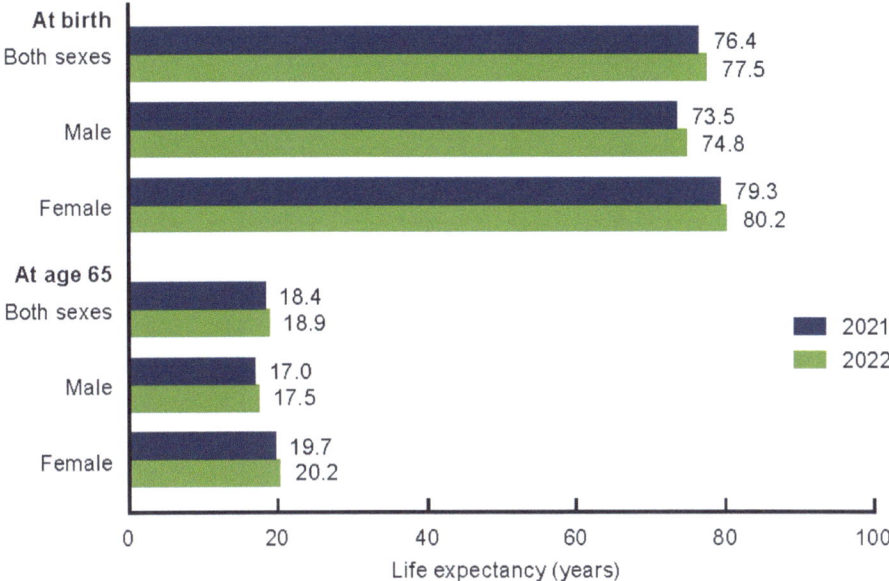

FIGURE 2-2 | Life expectancy at birth and age 65, by sex: United States, 2021 and 2022.
SOURCE: Kochanek et al., 2024.

TABLE 2-1 | Health Conditions Impacting Women and Men in the United States, 2022

Health Condition	Men (% having health condition in 2022)	Women (% having health condition in 2022)
COPD, emphysema, or chronic bronchitis	4.1	5.0
Asthma episode in the past 12 months	2.1	5.1
Any type of cancer	8.6	10.4
Arthritis	18.0	25.0
Obesity	32.8	33.5
Fair or poor health status	13.8	15.2
Did not get needed medical care due to cost in the past 12 months	5.4	7.1

NOTE: COPD = chronic obstructive pulmonary disease.
SOURCE: CDC NCHS, 2018.

as much per person"—and still experiences the highest infant and maternal mortality rates—more than three times as high as other wealthy countries (Gunja et al., 2022; Wagner et al., 2024). It should be noted that recent studies have questioned the validity of U.S. maternal mortality rates, attributing their elevation to issues with data reporting and aggregation, and noting that when adjusted for these data irregularities, they may be approximately equivalent to other wealthy countries (Simmons-Duffin, 2024). However, these studies also emphasize that even if these data are inaccurately reported and the overall rate is significantly lower, extreme disparities between ethnic and racial minorities are still present at alarming rates and must be addressed (Simmons-Duffin, 2024).

The U.S. maternal mortality rate for 2022 was lower than for 2021—22.3 deaths versus 32.9 per 100,000 live births, respectively—and maternal mortality rates for all groups decreased over this same period (Hoyert, 2024). However, the maternal mortality rate for non-Hispanic Black women in 2022 was 49.5 deaths per 100,000 live births, more than twice that of White women (19 per 100,000) and nearly three times that of Hispanic women (16.9 per 100,000) (Hoyert, 2024) (see Figure 2-3). In 2020, Norway's infant mortality rate was 1.6 deaths per 1,000

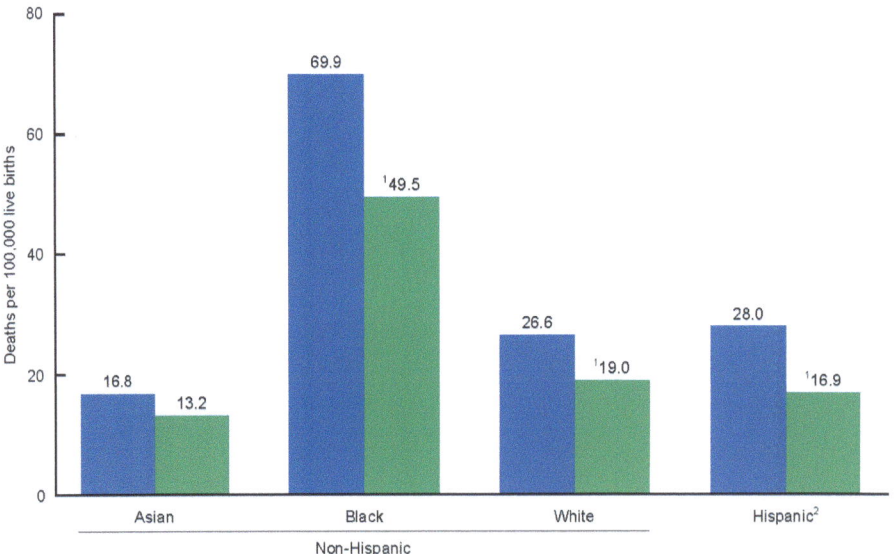

FIGURE 2-3 | Maternal mortality rate by race and Hispanic origin: United States, 2021 and 2022.
[1]Statistically significant decrease from previous year ($p < 0.05$).
[2]Hispanic people may be of any race.
NOTE: Race groups are single race.
SOURCE: Hoyert, 2024.

live births, while the United States experienced 5.4 deaths per 1,000 live births (Petrullo, 2023). In 2022, the Netherlands had the lowest maternal mortality rate of surveyed wealthy countries at 1.2 deaths per 100,000 live births, whereas the United States had 55.3 deaths per 100,000 live births (Gunja et al., 2022). High maternal death rates in the United States could be reversed by increasing access to primary care, providing comprehensive postpartum support, and implementing a "maternal health care workforce mainly comprising midwives covered by insurance" (Gunja et al., 2022, 2024).

Women comprise more than half of the U.S. population and experience overall worse health for more of their lives than men do, yet diseases that disproportionately impact this population are underfunded and understudied. Addressing these issues will not only significantly accelerate progress toward achieving health equity but is also a moral imperative in care for half of the American population.

Health Disparities Persist

Many health challenges affect subpopulations of the American public differently, a trend that has worsened in many disease areas despite concerted work to eliminate or ameliorate such disparities. This chapter touches on disparities related to gender, geographic location, and race/ethnicity but is in no way comprehensive. Chapter 4 of this publication examines health disparities—and the need for federal focus on their impacts—in greater detail.

Adults 35–64 who live in the American South and Midwest are currently dying at a higher rate than they were 40 years ago (Achenbach et al., 2023). There are many complex reasons for this increase, but they include a lack of comprehensive and high-quality health care—including having to travel long distances to access such care—and a prevalence of untreated or poorly treated chronic disease (Achenbach et al., 2023).

Health disparities along racial and ethnic lines plague almost every disease type but are most stark when the impacts of chronic diseases are considered. "American Indian/Alaska Native, Native Hawaiian and other Pacific Islander, and Black people [are] more than twice as likely as White people to die from diabetes, and Black people [are] more likely than White people to die from heart disease" (Hill et al., 2023). Health disparities not only impact the presence of disease but also impact their outcomes, as "[a]lthough Black people did not have higher cancer incidence rates than White people overall and across most types of cancer that were examined, they were more likely to die from cancer" (Hill et al., 2023). These stark health disparities show that the benefits of the U.S. biomedical research enterprise are not reaching all Americans equally. Historically marginalized and minoritized populations cannot continue to suffer disproportionately, and their care must be carefully planned and accounted for.

Deaths of Despair

Recent increases in early death rates among Americans—especially White Americans—are overwhelmingly due to deaths of despair, including mortality due to suicide, drug overdoses, and alcohol use (JEC, 2019).

Deaths by suicide increased from 10.4 deaths per 100,000 in 2000 to 14.1 per 100,000 in 2021—accounting for more than 48,000 Americans per year (CDC, 2024b). Health disparities are also present in deaths by suicide because American Indian/Alaska Native and White individuals are the most likely to die by suicide compared to other racial and ethnic groups—28.1 individuals per 100,000 and 17.4 per 100,000, respectively. Men were also 4.5 times more likely to die by suicide than women were in 2021 (Garnett and Curtin, 2023) (see Figure 2-4).

Drug overdose deaths in the United States have increased drastically across all populations in the past 20 years and have doubled in the past decade (NIH NIDA, 2024). Notably, overdose deaths decreased by 3% in 2023 compared to 2022, but an excess of 100,000 preventable deaths is by no means a success (CDC NCHS, 2024). Deaths related to opioids—primarily fentanyl—decreased, but deaths due to cocaine and methamphetamine increased, signaling, potentially, a new area of necessary focus (CDC NCHS, 2024).

"Deaths due to excessive alcohol use, including partially and fully alcohol-attributable conditions, increased … 29% between 2016 and 2021" (Esser et al., 2024). Although alcohol-related deaths among men are more common—119,606 deaths in 2020–2021—rates of death among women increased more dramatically—from 43,565 in 2016 to 58,701 in 2021, or a 35% increase (Esser et al., 2024).

The types of mortality that compose the deaths of despair are, by their nature, complex—including biological and mental components—and are heavily influenced by the social determinants of health. The U.S. biomedical research enterprise will, more likely than not, be unable to invent a drug or single therapy to address deaths of despair. A coordinated, strategic approach to each type of mortality will be necessary to reverse these trends and prevent their recurrence.

Obesity

Worldwide obesity has tripled since 1975 (WHO, 2024). In the late 1980s, about 20% of U.S. adults older than 20 had a body mass index (BMI) of 30 or higher, which defines them as obese according to the World Health Organization

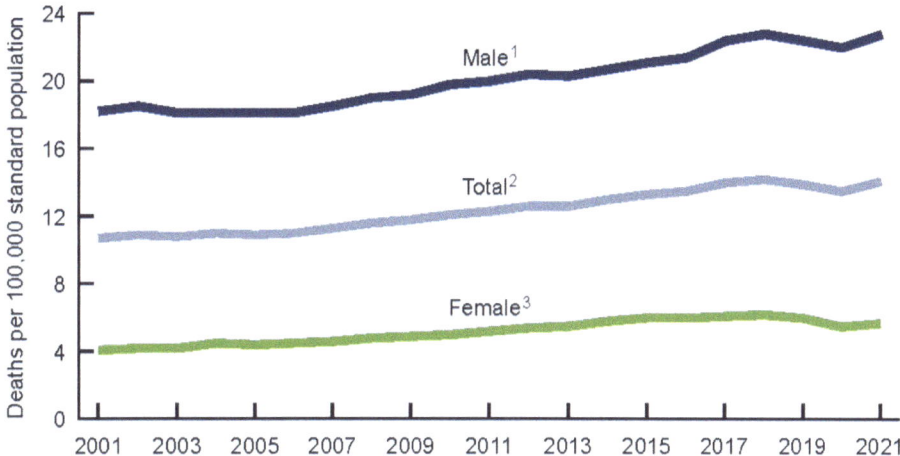

FIGURE 2-4 | Age-adjusted suicide rates by sex: United States, 2001–2021.
[1]No statistically significant trend from 2001 through 2006; significant increasing trend from 2006 to 2018; no statistically significant trend from 2018 through 2021, $p < 0.05$. The rate in 2021 was significantly higher than the rate in 2020, $p < 0.05$.
[2]No statistically significant trend from 2001 through 2006; significant increasing trend from 2006 to 2018, with different rates of change over time; no statistically significant trend from 2018 through 2021, $p < 0.05$. The rate in 2021 was significantly higher than the rate in 2020, $p < 0.05$.
[3]Significant increasing trend from 2001 to 2017; significant decreasing trend from 2017 through 2021, $p < 0.05$. The rate in 2021 was significantly higher than the rate in 2020, $p < 0.05$.
NOTES: Suicide deaths are identified using *International Classification of Diseases, 10th Revision* underlying cause-of-death codes U03, X60–X84, and Y87.0. Age-adjusted death rates are calculated using the direct method and the 2000 U.S. standard population. Access data table for Figure 1 at https://www.cdc.gov/nchs/data/databriefs/db464-tables.pdf#1.
SOURCE: Garnett and Curtin, 2023.

(WHO, 2024). As of 2018, 42%—or twice as many—of U.S. adults have a BMI of 30 or higher, and the trend appears to be increasing (NIH NIDDK, 2021). Additionally, childhood obesity has become increasingly dire in the United States, where 1 in 5 children and adolescents have obesity (CDC, 2024c). Obesity is an especially complex condition because it is caused by an interconnected and inextricable web of factors, including food intake, lack of physical activity, sleep habits, socioeconomic status, geographic location, and other social determinants of health (NIH NIDDK, 2021). Such a complex condition requires the input of many experts from a variety of fields—a strong argument for the necessity of a coordinated national strategic vision and a convergence science approach.

Diseases of Aging

More Americans are living longer, and the size of the population of baby boomers, in particular, will add to the number of diseases of aging appearing and being treated—especially dementias including Alzheimer's disease (Knickman and Snell, 2002). In 2017, more than 250,000 deaths were attributed to dementia, and 50% of those deaths were attributed to Alzheimer's disease (Kramarow and Tejada-Vera, 2019). As of 2021, 6.2 million Americans over 65 are living with Alzheimer's disease, which is estimated to grow to 13.8 million by 2060 (No author, 2022b). While deaths from cardiovascular disease and HIV have decreased, deaths due to Alzheimer's disease have increased by more than 145% since 2000 (No author, 2021) (see Figure 2-5). Aging is the biggest risk factor for Alzheimer's disease, and it doubles every 5 years over the age of 65 (Brookmeyer et al., 2011). Living longer is not meaningful unless the extra years lived are healthful, and as such, diseases of aging demand the attention of the U.S. biomedical research enterprise.

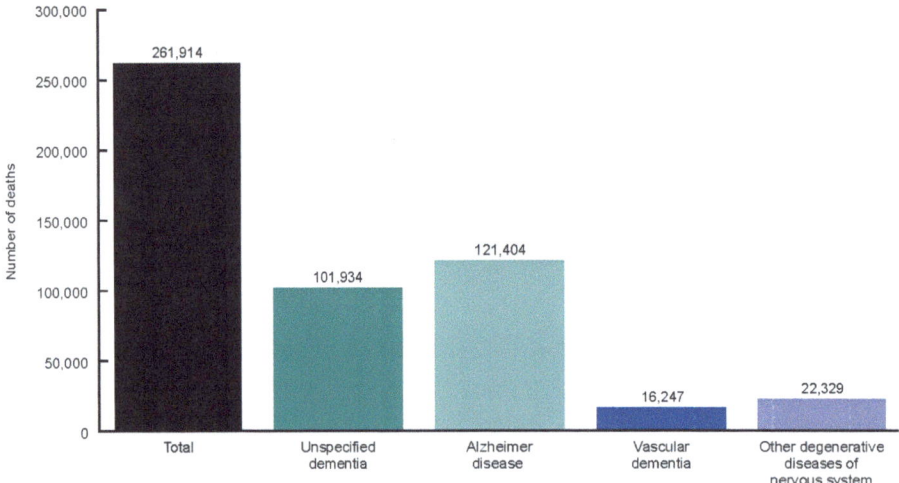

FIGURE 2-5 | U.S. deaths due to dementias.
NOTE: Dementia deaths are identified according to the *International Classification of Diseases, 10th Revision* underlying cause-of-death codes: F03 (unspecified dementia), G30 (Alzheimer's disease), F01 (vascular dementia), and G31 (other degenerative diseases of nervous system).
SOURCE: Kramarow and Tejada-Vera, 2019.

The Next Pandemic

The probability of facing another pandemic with COVID-19-level impact—which cost the world trillions of dollars and more than 7 million lives—was recently estimated at 1 in 50 in any given year (CEPI, 2024; Worldometer, 2024). This means that an individual's chance of experiencing another pandemic over their lifetime is approximately 38% (CEPI, 2024). With hundreds of emerging or re-emerging pathogens affecting human health and hundreds of thousands of uncatalogued pathogens in existence, this is a crucial moment to strengthen the biomedical research enterprise for health security nationally and globally. Biomedical research is critical for tracking, preventing, addressing, and mitigating another such calamity, as well as ensuring that scientific infrastructure and person-power can be leveraged to avoid human suffering.

Climate Change

Climate change is a looming environmental threat as well as an urgent public health threat, because millions of people die every year due to health issues related to climate change (NAM, 2024). Climate change can exacerbate existing diseases and create new ones, including "respiratory and heart diseases, Lyme disease, West Nile virus, water- and food-related illnesses, and injuries and deaths" (EPA, 2024). By its very nature, climate change requires a convergence science approach to address its root causes and reverse its multiple cascading effects.

PUBLIC TRUST IS CRITICAL FOR THE ACCEPTANCE OF A NATIONAL STRATEGIC VISION

The American public has recently shown a significant mistrust of science and public health officials—a disturbing trend that, if prolonged, will likely negatively impact the nation's health. Even if the U.S. biomedical research enterprise produces revolutionary and life-saving treatments, if the public does not trust science and medicine and will not accept the treatments, then the effort will have been for naught.

Beyond general trust in science, patient engagement is also critical for the success of the U.S. health care system—with the added benefit of directly leading to improved outcomes for patients and their clinicians (Marzban et al., 2022). Patient engagement is an ethical practice—reflecting the "nothing about us without us" principle that has guided disability activism—and a powerful path to meaningful scientific progress and improved health outcomes for all (United

Nations Enable, 2004). Progress in improving health over the years has wholly depended on public trust and patient engagement—and, specifically, enough public trust and patient engagement for individuals to actively participate in clinical trials. Experimental treatments cannot advance without such partnership. To achieve the levels of engagement and participation needed to advance science and medicine, the public must trust science and scientists.

Shawn Otto, author of *The War on Science*, reviewed the history of science and public trust and has asserted that funding for science after the Second World War caused scientists to turn inward, cultivating the scientific community and not engaging the public as they had before the war (Otto, 2016). The result, he says, was that the public discourse around science, including the politicization of science, largely did not include scientists themselves. Otto reflected on this time, "[s]cience creates knowledge—knowledge is power, and that power is political" (Otto, 2016). Science has, in 2024, become so complex that few members of the lay public can appreciate the challenges of the practice or the value of the outputs, which often leads to fear and mistrust. Mistrust is exacerbated by intentional misdirection or manipulation—often amplified by social media—as well as current challenges with reproducibility in scientific and medical experiments (Kington et al., 2021; NASEM, 2019a).

According to The Pew Research Center, which has been measuring public trust in science for more than 20 years, most Americans are still more confident that scientists and clinicians are acting in the public's best interest than other groups are, but that confidence has fallen since COVID-19 (Kennedy and Tyson, 2023). In 2020, 89% of American adults had a great deal or a fair amount of confidence in clinicians to act in the best interests of the public, with 11% having not too much or no confidence at all (Kennedy and Tyson, 2023). Since then, survey results show that confidence in clinicians has fallen by 8% and scientists by 14%, with a reciprocal increase of about one-quarter of American adults having not too much or no confidence at all that clinicians or scientists act in the best interests of the public (see Figure 2-6).

When asked whether science has had a positive or negative impact on society, the share of adult Americans who believe it has been a net positive has also declined since 2020, and the share who believe it has been a net negative has more than doubled from 3% in 2019 to 8% in 2023 (Kennedy and Tyson, 2023). More concerning is how these views differ across racial and ethnic groups, and how they may directly influence the outsized health inequities described throughout this Special Publication. More than 50% of White and Asian Americans say science has had a mostly positive impact on society, whereas that sentiment is held by less than 50% of Black and Hispanic Americans (see Figure 2-7). In

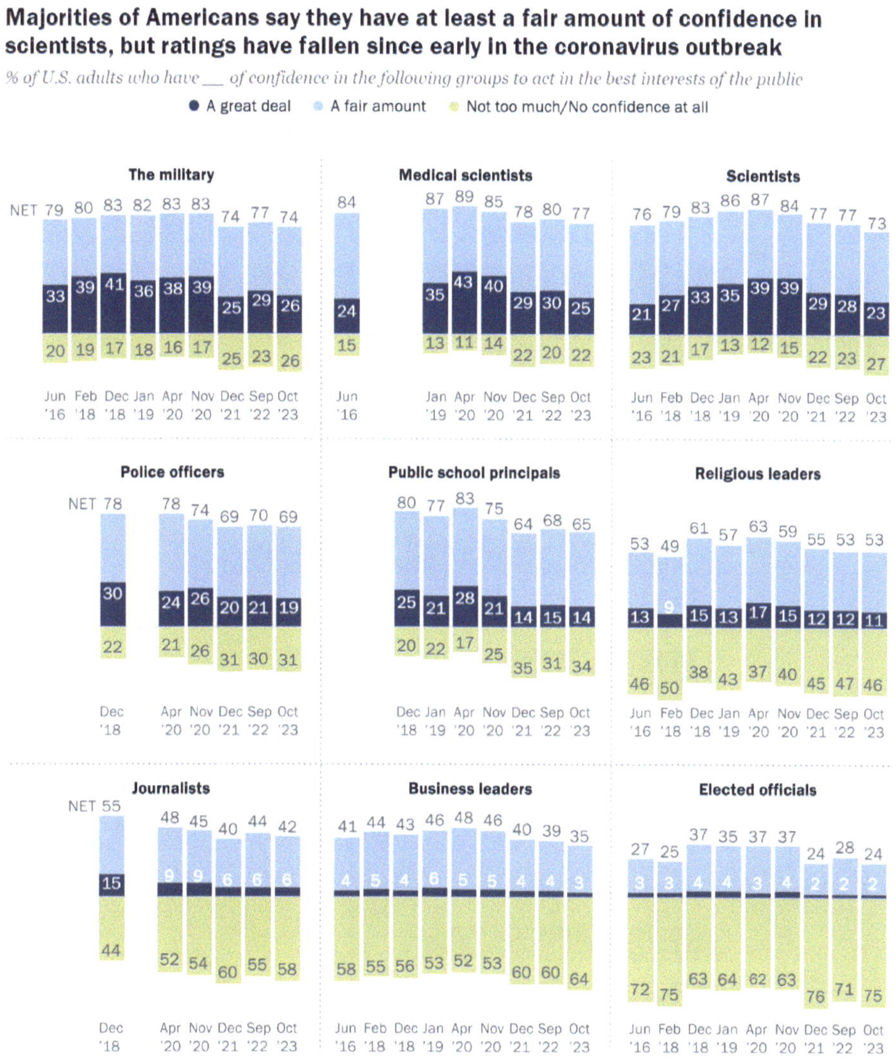

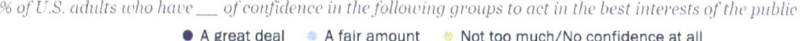

FIGURE 2-6 | American confidence in scientists falls.
NOTE: Respondents who did not give an answer are not shown.
SOURCE: Kennedy and Tyson, 2023.

addition, positive views on the effect of science on society increase with the level of education. Among individuals with a high school education or less, only 42% say science is a net positive, whereas 72% of those with college degrees say science is a net positive (Kennedy and Tyson, 2023). As noted, these trends likely contribute to health and health care disparities and should be addressed

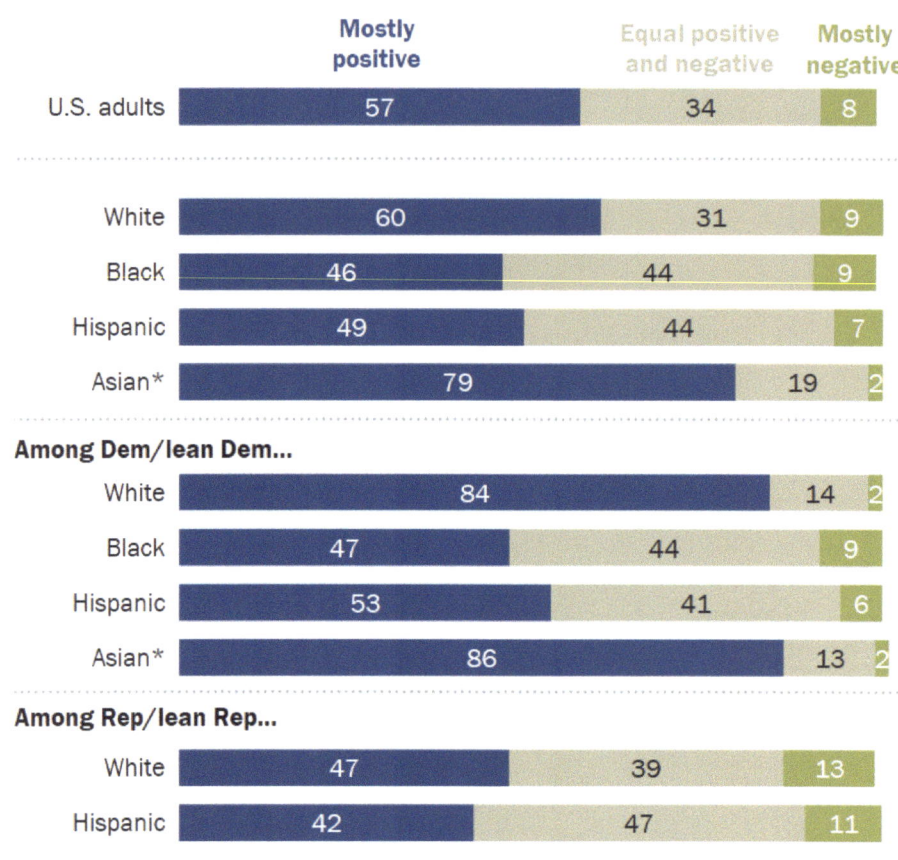

FIGURE 2-7 | Trust in science varies among groups.
* Estimates for Asian adults are representative of English speakers only.
NOTES: Survey of U.S. adults conducted September 25–October 1, 2023. Sample sizes for Black and Asian Republicans are too small to analyze responses separately. Respondents who did not give an answer are not shown. White, Black, and Asian adults include those who report being only one race and are non-Hispanic. Hispanic adults are of any race.
SOURCE: Kennedy and Tyson, 2023.

to increase necessary representation in health science research, which will help improve health outcomes for all.

Given its enormous influence on biomedical research, NIH should work to ensure that the U.S. biomedical research enterprise continues to embrace and actively pursue improved patient engagement. As part of this effort, NIH leadership should continue to prioritize the National Library of Medicine's efforts to modernize the clinical trials clearinghouse located at https://www.clinicaltrials.gov. This modernization process, which has been informed by broad engagement with patients and other members of the research community, will meaningfully improve both patients' and providers' experiences in seeking opportunities to participate in clinical research (NIH NLM, 2023). NIH should also focus on expanding platforms that support collaboration with the patient community, including those hosted by the Patient-Centered Outcomes Research Institute (PCORI) and Clinical and Translational Science Awards (NIH NCATS, 2024; PCORI, n.d.).

Although the history of engaging non-scientists in NIH advisory panels and other patient engagement efforts is long, a full embrace of public engagement in biomedical research remains a work in progress and requires a strong foundation of trust on which to grow (NIH, n.d.a). Work in this area should include not only a rigorous commitment to elevating patient voices in research but also efforts to foster meaningful trust-building and improved communication between scientists and the public they serve. Prioritizing public trust to enhance patient engagement is critical for advancing biomedical research in the United States.

MORE EFFECTIVE CLINICAL TRIALS WILL BENEFIT ALL RESEARCH

A healthy person with low trust in science and scientists could certainly carry that mistrust into their own medical journey if faced with serious illness or life-threatening health challenges, and that mistrust would likely lead to challenging engagement with the health system. Patient engagement in the United States is inconsistent at best, and if improved would expand trust and might also accelerate the development of new treatments. Patients play a critical role in the design and execution of research by participating in clinical trials for promising new drugs and other treatments. Early data from PCORI suggest that involving patients throughout the clinical research process—including study design, conduct, and dissemination of results—leads to improved research that focuses on topics important to patients, maximizes their participation, decreases patient and provider burden, enhances enrollment, and improves data quality (Forsythe et al., 2019).

Adequate and diverse clinical trial participation continues to vex NIH and industry partners alike because recruiting and retaining participants remains a challenge. According to one pharmaceutical executive, less than 5% of eligible patients participate in clinical trials, 30% of those who do enroll drop out, and 20% of trial sites fail to enroll patients at all (Smalley, 2018). A study published in 2021 reported that "convenience-enhancing" solutions such as transportation arrangements, child care, and the use of mobile apps may meaningfully increase patient engagement in clinical trials, particularly among underrepresented populations (Sine et al., 2021). This study reveals an important lesson—that patient concerns about participating in research are not solely about scientific approaches or clinical settings. In addition to a diagnosis, people bring their personal circumstances, knowledge, and preferred ways to receive and manage their medical information to all interactions with the health care system and the biomedical research enterprise. Acknowledging the whole person—not just the patient's disease—will likely generate greater trust between scientists and clinical trial participants.

Relatedly, challenges surrounding patient engagement are often framed as a communications gap, when scientific experts describing their research fail to connect with patients. In reality, this disconnect is about more than language—patients need researchers to acknowledge and support the value of the patient in all stages of research and development.

The COVID-19 pandemic caused many in-person clinical trial sites to shut down and gave rise to an increase in decentralized trials. These trials rely less on frequent, in-person office visits by using mobile apps and virtual and digital platforms to track data, symptoms, and outcomes and conduct interventions when needed (Hanley et al., 2023). Decentralized trials, which have been in development for years but were slowly adopted until they were necessary in 2020, have the potential to remove many barriers to broader participation.

There is a need for more Americans in general to participate in clinical trials, but there is a particularly urgent need to diversify clinical trial cohorts. To produce generalizable results and ensure the safety and efficacy of novel drugs and treatments, a clinical trial cohort must reflect the composition of the population it is intended to serve, and America's current clinical trial structure and recruiting approaches do not support or ensure this diversity (Acuña-Villaorduña et al., 2023). A National Academies consensus study found that a lack of progress on this issue could compromise the generalizability of research to the entire U.S. population, cost hundreds of billions of dollars in decreased life expectancy and years in the labor force, and may impede discoveries, among other impacts (NASEM, 2022). Diversity in clinical trial cohorts could be improved in several ways, all of which require a reimagining and restructuring of how clinical trials are executed. A low-effort intervention is suggested by the finding that, despite a pervasive belief among biomedical researchers that underrepresented populations do not want to participate in clinical trials, these populations are "no less likely, and in some cases are more likely, to participate in research *if they are asked*" (emphasis added) (NASEM, 2022). Ensuring the participation of racial and ethnic minorities and individuals who live in rural areas is of outsized importance to appropriate cohort diversity and "effective delivery of potentially efficacious investigational therapies to patients … without other available treatment options" (Acuña-Villaorduña et al., 2023). Novel approaches to solve these pervasive issues could include embedding clinical trials within communities, rather than locating them at large hospitals or academic medical centers, which are disproportionately located in large cities; providing additional funding to assist participants with the expenses of participating in a clinical trial; and broadly employing and utilizing patient navigators (Acuña-Villaorduña et al., 2023). Expanding pools of clinical trial participants and ensuring that they are representative of the actual composition of the population the intervention is intended to serve will require a sea change in how clinical trials are imagined, structured, and executed, but will ultimately help to move all biomedical research forward more expeditiously.

GLOBAL BEST PRACTICES AND LESSONS LEARNED

Despite the United States' long leadership in biomedical research, over the past few decades, other nations have started to invest more heavily in their own research efforts. Although the United States continues to spend more in absolute dollars, other nations are now investing a greater percentage of their GDP in R&D than the United States does (see Figure 2-8). U.S. federal investment in biomedical research has mostly remained level since 2010 when accounting for inflation.

Many of America's peer nations have enacted long-term strategic plans for science and technology that couple with and support their increased financial investments. China's first 12-year plan was the Long-term Plan for the Development of Science and Technology 1956–1967 (Embassy of the People's Republic of China in the Hellenic Republic, 2004). Its most recent plan—the 15-year Medium- to Long-Term Plan for the Development of Science and Technology—includes goals to invest 2.5% of its GDP in R&D, limit its dependence on imported technology, increase the overall number of patents, and have "Chinese-authored scientific papers [be] among the world's most cited" (Cao et al., 2006) (see Box 2-2). In 1995, Japan enacted its Science and Technology Basic Law and then established strategic plans every 5 years (NRC, 2009). Its most recent plan aims to improve access to data for all of its citizens; collaboratively address global issues such as

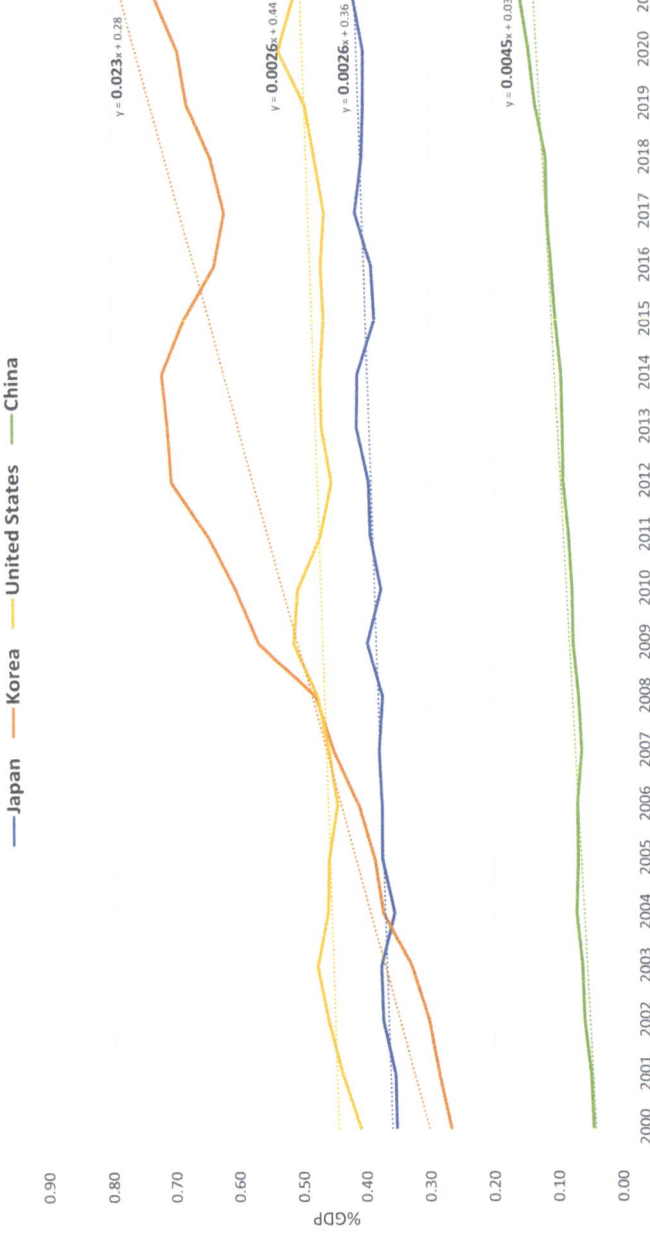

FIGURE 2-8 | Basic science research expenditures (% gross domestic product) by country, 2000–2021.

NOTES: Each line represents expenditures for basic science research as a percentage of gross domestic product (GDP) for each country, where each country is represented by different colored lines. Dotted lines indicate linear trends over time, with corresponding equations shown above each trend line. Research expenditures include all research and are not limited to biomedical research. Parameters for the data shown in Figure 2-8 within the Main Science and Technology Indicators database are as follows: time period = 2000–2021; reference areas = South Korea, United States, China, and Japan; measure = basic science research expenditure; and unit of measure = percentage GDP.
SOURCE: OECD, n.d.b.

climate change and COVID-19; and build a "resilient, safe, and secure society" (Government of Japan, 2021). Singapore created its National Technology Plan in 1991 to "steer the development of science and technology … [and] enhance [its] economic competitiveness" (Ministry of Trade and Industry Singapore, 2006). Its most recent plan includes broadening the scope of research to address emerging needs, expanding the nation's research base in terms of topics and funding, and driving technology translation (National Research Foundation, Prime Minister's Office Singapore, n.d.) (see Box 2-1). The European Union's strategy for 2020–2024 focuses on environment and climate, the digital future, jobs and economy, "protecting our citizens and our values," Europe in the world, and democracy and rights (European Commission, 2020) (see Box 2-3).

As America's peer nations continue to scale up their investment—in funding and person-power—in biomedical research and utilize strategic planning to guide these major investments, it follows that the United States would be well served to follow suit. The U.S. national strategic vision should draw from the successes and best practices established by our peer nations, and three key examples are outlined in Boxes 2-1, 2-2, and 2-3 below.

BOX 2-1

National Agenda Setting Example 1: Singapore

In 2000, the Singaporean government, motivated to increase its knowledge capital, established a National Biomedical Science Strategy. This Strategy established A*STAR—the Agency for Science, Technology and Research—under the Ministry of Trade and Industry and in 2003, opened Biopolis, a biomedical R&D hub (*Science*, 2007). The number of Singapore-based biotech companies increased from 7 in 2012 to 52 in 2022, and large international pharmaceutical companies, such as Sanofi, BioNTech, and Merck have established local offices in Singapore (Weidong, 2024). Furthermore, Duke University and the National University of Singapore collaborated to open a new medical school, Duke-NUS (DukeNUS Medical School, 2022).

Singapore's biomedical science manufacturing output increased from $6 billion in 2000 to $29.4 billion in 2012 (Antara, 2013). During the same period, employment in biomedical science grew from 6,000 to 15,700 (Antara, 2013). As of 2019, Singapore's biomedical manufacturing sector represents 4% of its total GDP (Whellams, 2021). Between 2000 and 2020, Singapore invested $10 billion into R&D and its current Research, Innovation and Enterprise 2025 strategic plan includes $19 billion in government funding (Tan, 2021).

BOX 2-2
National Agenda Setting Example 2: China

Launched in 2006 by China's State Council, the Medium- and Long-Term Plan for the Development of Science and Technology 2006–2020 (MLP) aimed to achieve four goals:"increase the nation's expenditure on R&D to 2.5% GDP, increase the contribution of science and technology progress to economic growth from less than 40% to more than 60%, reduce dependence on foreign technology to 30% or less, and become one of the top five countries in terms of number of invention patents and manuscript citations" (Cao et al., 2006).

China has directed its national science and technology 5-year plans, which have existed since 1953, toward achieving MLP goals. Additionally, China prioritized funding for 16 "mega-engineering programs"—covering topics such as circuit manufacturing, oil and gas exploration, drug development, smart grid, big data, and health security—and four "mega-science programs"—including a deep-sea space station, quantum computing, and brain science—as funding priorities (Sun and Cao, 2021). The MLP aimed to address challenges that arose from decentralization of R&D spending, which Sun and Cao say resulted from a lack of top-level design, unified planning, and coordination (Sun and Cao, 2021). Through its national science and technology programs, China reconfigured its public funding system to align basic, applied, and development research with 3- to 5-year timelines.

China achieved all targets set by the last MLP. By 2020, China was investing 2.4% of GDP into R&D, just shy of its 2.5% goal (Sun and Cao, 2021). By 2019 the contribution of science and technology progress to economic growth bloomed from 40% to 59.5%, just shy of its 60% goal (Sun and Cao, 2021). An original goal was to reduce dependence on foreign technology to 30% or less, but China stopped using this measure in 2016. However, in that same year China reduced its dependence to 31.2%, just shy of the initial goal (Sun and Cao, 2021). Lastly, in 2018, China ranked third globally for triadic patents and second globally for manuscript citations (Sun and Cao, 2021).

China has since launched its new Medium- and Long-Term Science and Technology Development Plan 2021–2035. However, unlike previous plans, the current plan has not been publicly released (Cheung et al., 2022).

BOX 2-3
National Agenda Setting Example 3: European Union

The Framework Programmes for Research and Technological Development were launched in 1984 as 5-year funding cycles to foster and coordinate research across the European Research Area (SERI, n.d.). In 2014, the cycle length was extended to 7 years and renamed Horizon 2020. The budget for the current Horizon Europe 2021–2027 is €95.5 billion (European Commission, 2021a). Horizon Europe aims to tackle climate change, boost European Union growth and innovation, support knowledge creation, and create new jobs and technologies (European Commission, 2021a). About one quarter of the Horizon Europe plan is dedicated to "excellent science." Of the approximately €25 billion earmarked for excellent science, €16 billion will be competitively funded to support investigator research through The European Research Council; €6.6 billion will fund doctoral education and postdoctoral and visiting scholar training through Marie Sklodowska-Curie Actions; and €2.4 billion will be directed toward integrating and improving research infrastructures across Europe (European Commission, 2021b). Under a separate pillar aimed at boosting European industrial competitiveness, €8.25 billion is dedicated to "generating new knowledge, developing innovative solutions and integrating where relevant a gender perspective to prevent, diagnose, monitor, treat and cure diseases" as well as developing health technologies; mitigating health risks; protecting populations; promoting good health and well-being; making public health systems more cost-effective, equitable, and sustainable; preventing and tackling poverty-related diseases; and supporting and enabling patient participation and self-management (European Commission, 2021c).

A robust evaluation system measuring success across three performance indicators is central to the success of Horizon Europe. The three performance indicators are scientific impact that includes creating high-quality new knowledge, strengthening human capital, and fostering dissemination and open science; economic impact that encompasses business creation and growth that will create direct and indirect jobs; and societal impact that addresses European Union priorities and global challenges, including United Nations Sustainable Development Goals (European Commission, 2023).

As of 2024, Horizon 2020 funded more than 35,000 projects that resulted in more than 4,000 patents and trademarks, grew employment by 20%, produced 276,000 peer-reviewed publications, supported 33 Nobel Prize winners, and provided 24,000 researchers globally with access to Europe's research infrastructure (European Commission, 2024).

CALL TO ACTION

The U.S. biomedical research enterprise is currently limited by fragmented research agendas dictated primarily by funding source rather than by strategic national public health needs. Despite spending more on R&D than any other nation, research expenditures in America are driven not by a national mission to improve health, but by motivations such as marketability and profit margins, which likely do not serve the nation's most pressing needs.

Relatedly, the federal government's current process of launching new initiatives in parallel or under the umbrellas of specific agencies decentralizes and diffuses national priorities. As multidisciplinary biomedical research and convergence science become more integral to all scientific progress, a coordinating and vision-setting body that sits above all federal agencies with the power to set strategy, provide guidance on resource allocation, and receive input from a broad variety of stakeholders is necessary to guide the U.S. biomedical research enterprise of the future.

The development and work of this advisory body should be informed by the vision-setting bodies of other nations—especially how they set strategy and coordinate funding to maximize efficiency and minimize redundancy. As other nations focus the efforts of their biomedical research enterprises with careful strategic planning, dedicate increasing amounts of their GDP to their enterprises, and work to become leaders in biomedical research, the United States should develop and deploy its own comprehensive strategy to maintain global leadership in biomedical research.

To achieve this vision, the authors of this Special Publication propose the following:

Priority 1-1: A U.S. biomedical research enterprise advisory body, created by the President of the United States and Congress, to galvanize national leadership, develop a national strategic vision, and coordinate efforts and resources.

Priority 1-2: This advisory body could:
- Be composed of leading scientists from a wide variety of disciplines, such as life, physical, social, and behavioral sciences; engineering; economics; and the humanities to ensure a convergence science approach to addressing all emerging needs;
- Engage with multiple relevant federal agencies;
- Be established with long terms;

- Be empowered to set national goals and benchmarks;
- Provide input on resource allocation that matches strategy;
- Consider, examine, and utilize global best practices in all aspects of its work, but especially as guidance for developing the national strategic vision;
- Include patients, caregivers, and members of the public to provide transparency and public engagement;
- Have clear, measurable goals and timelines;
- Coordinate with the National Economic Policy Council and the Domestic Policy Council to ensure the engagement of all relevant stakeholders; and
- Monitor their progress and report to Congress and the American public annually on their work.

Priority 1-3: The advisory body's national strategic vision could:
- Directly address the current fragmentation in funding and agenda-setting present in the U.S. biomedical research enterprise, in concert with the efforts proposed in Priorities 4-1 and 4-2. The national strategic vision cannot succeed without coordination and alignment of funding and agenda-setting, which, conversely, cannot be coordinated and aligned without the guidance of a national strategic vision. These Priorities cannot be separated.
- Set priorities for the use of convergence science and implement a roadmap for bringing together relevant agencies and scientific disciplines to achieve this collaborative approach (see also Priority 4-2).
- Consider and propose funding to address:
  - Existing and emerging health challenges, including but not limited to infant and maternal mortality, women's health concerns, deaths of despair, obesity, climate change, health disparities, diseases with pandemic potential, and diseases of aging;
  - Future health threats such as increasing risks of extreme heat and other natural disasters due to climate change and emerging or existing infectious diseases;
  - Public engagement in the entire U.S. biomedical research enterprise, but especially focused on increased participation in clinical trials;
  - Deteriorating public trust in science and medicine;
  - Prioritization and development of new and innovative research approaches to reduce and eliminate health disparities; and
  - The needs of the U.S. biomedical research enterprise workforce, including adjusting historical pathways to employment or tenure as emerging health challenges, approaches to science, or the needs of the American public change.

3
STREAMLINED, COORDINATED, AND INCREASINGLY IMPACTFUL FUNDING

According to the National Science Board's Science & Engineering Indicators, global research and development (R&D) expenditures have grown from $726 billion in 2000 to $2.4 trillion in 2019 (Burke et al., 2022). The United States is the global leader in gross domestic expenditure on R&D with $656 billion in 2019, accounting for 27% of the global total (Burke et al., 2022). In the same year, China accounted for 22% of the global total with $526 billion; therefore, China and the United States alone account for half of all global R&D. Other countries with significant gross expenditures on R&D include Japan, Germany, and South Korea (Burke et al., 2022).

In 2019, the United States spent more than 3% of its $21.4 trillion gross domestic product (GDP) on R&D and absolute spending on R&D has increased from $268 billion in 2000 to $656 billion in 2019 (Burke et al., 2022). While the United States spends the most globally in absolute dollars on R&D, other countries have started to invest a greater percentage of their GDPs in R&D than the United States does (see Figure 3-1). China has increased its percentage of GDP spending at nearly two times the rate of the United States (see Figure 3-1) and South Korea is spending 5% of its GDP on R&D—second only to Israel at 5.56% (Investopedia, 2024; World Bank, 2023). Basic research expenditures as a percentage of GDP mirror patterns of total research expenditures, with South Korea showing the greatest increase between 2000 and 2021, followed by China and the United States, while Japan has seen much less growth (see Figure 3-2).

Funding is not everything when it comes to biomedical research, but it does enable continuous, focused, and innovative research. The United States has long been a global leader in biomedical research—partially due to large financial investments—but the trends described above show that the rest of the globe is

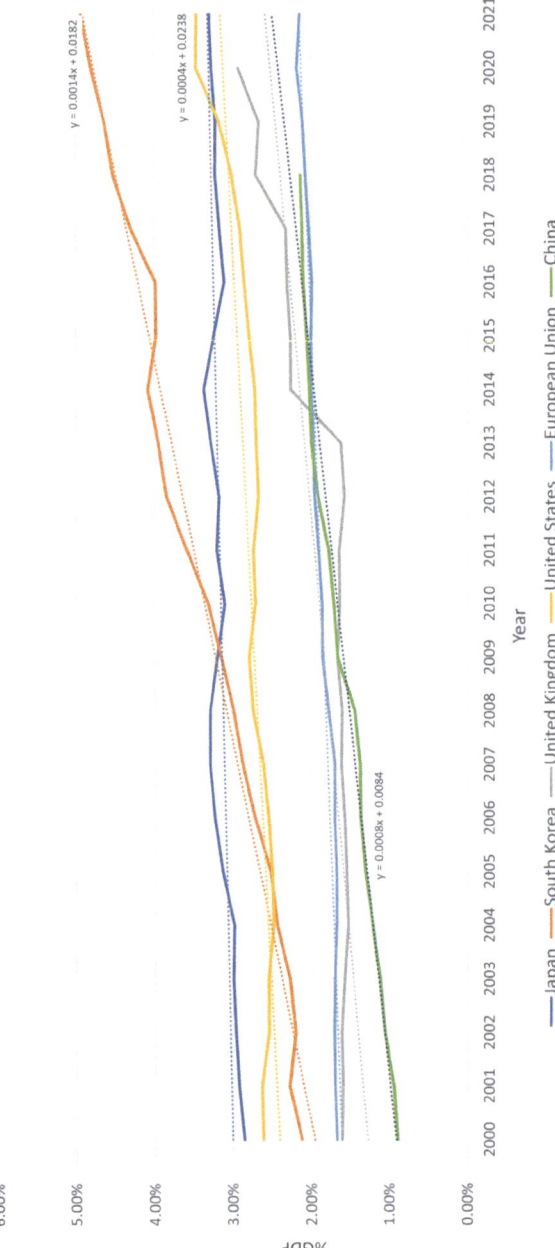

FIGURE 3-1 | Gross expenditures on research and development by country, in terms of % gross domestic product, 2000–2021.
SOURCE: OECD, n.d.c.

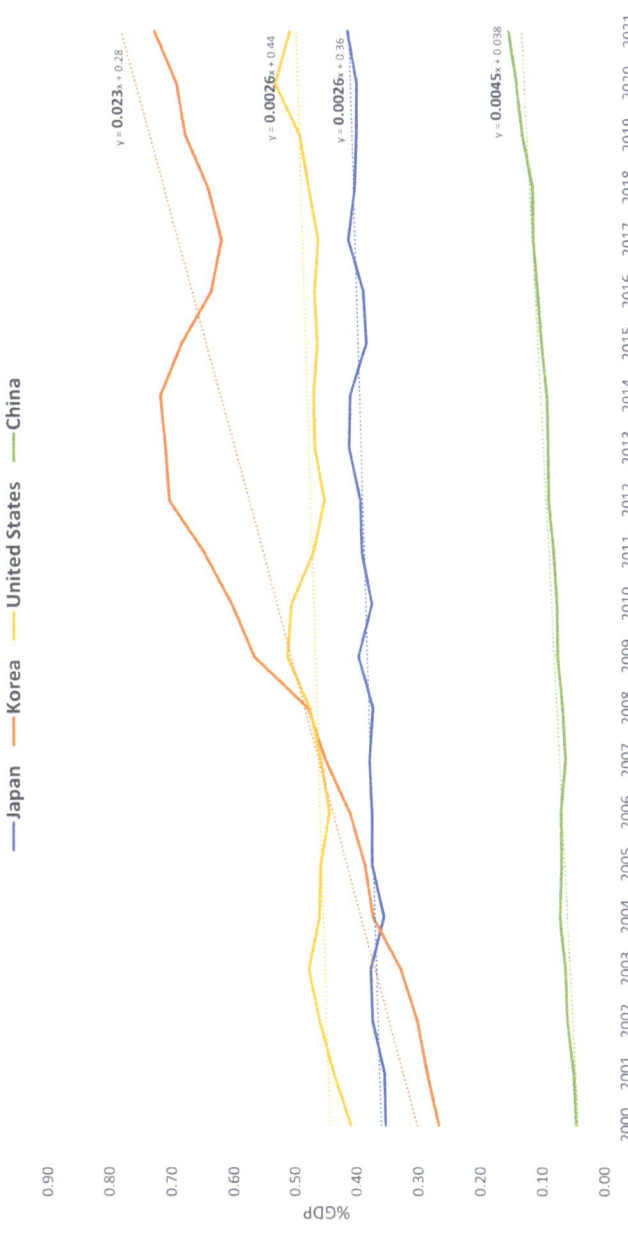

FIGURE 3-2 | Basic science research expenditures (% gross domestic product) by country, 2000–2021.
NOTES: Dotted lines indicate linear trends over time, with corresponding equations shown above each trend line. Research expenditures include all research and are not limited to biomedical research. China's basic science research expenditures are increasing at a rate of 0.0045% gross domestic product (GDP) per year, while the United States and Japan's basic science research expenditures are increasing at a rate of 0.0026% GDP per year and South Korea's are increasing at a rate of 0.023% GDP per year. Parameters for the data shown in Figure 3-2 within the Main Science and Technology Indicators database are as follows: time period = 2000–2021; reference areas = South Korea, United States, China, and Japan; measure = basic science research expenditure; and unit of measure = percentage GDP.
SOURCE: OECD, n.d.b.

catching up. To continue to enable American breakthroughs and maintain global leadership, the sources, coordination, and disbursement of funding across the U.S. biomedical research enterprise should be examined.

FUNDING ALWAYS COMES WITH AN AGENDA

Many, if not all, of America's scientific breakthroughs were enabled by large financial investments. The U.S. biomedical research enterprise is driven by federal funding, mostly through the National Institutes of Health (NIH), but is also supported by funding from industry, venture capital, and philanthropy. Each of these funding sources arrives with an agenda and is very rarely "no strings attached." The somewhat piecemeal funding apparatus of the U.S. biomedical research enterprise and these competing agendas are barriers to a truly coordinated system, where initiatives to solve complex problems are launched in concert instead of in parallel and funding is focused on where it will have the largest impact.

"Venture capital funding drives the biotechnology industry, but money is the main driver of venture capital," James Flynn, managing partner at Deerfield Management Company, said when he spoke to the authors of the Special Publication. Deerfield is an investment firm focused on life science research, medical device development, diagnostics, digital health, and health services (Deerfield, n.d.). To Flynn's point, organizations such as Deerfield are driven by one main obligation—providing returns to their investors (Zider, 1998). This focus requires venture capital firms to seek clear value propositions and greatly limit their risk, which narrows the aperture of the number and type of projects and science they are comfortable supporting. Investor expectations of receiving returns on investment also preclude full incorporation of venture capital endeavors into existing R&D funding models (Zider, 1998).

Like venture capital, industry spending is also driven by expectations of profit. While the U.S. government is the largest single investor in biomedical research, private industry as a sector is the largest overall investor, spending more than double the NIH budget in 2019 on development and bringing products to market (Research!America and Teconomy Partners, LLC, 2022). Despite industry's significant investments in biomedical research, its focus is mostly on products rather than discovery research (Research!America and Teconomy Partners, LLC, 2022). According to a recent report published by the Deloitte Centre for Health Solutions, the 20 pharmaceutical companies that spend the most on R&D spent a total of $139 billion in 2022, a slight decrease from the high of $141 billion in 2021 (Deloitte Centre for Health Solutions, 2023). The average cost of bringing a drug to market was $1.9 billion in 2021 and $2.2 billion in 2022 (Deloitte Centre for Health Solutions, 2023).

Deloitte reports that internal rates of return from R&D investment have been declining for the past decade, and several factors contribute to these decreased margins—most notably the increasing duration of clinical trials (Deloitte Centre for Health Solutions, 2023). The average time span of a clinical trial from the start of Phase I to the end of Phase III has grown longer in the last decade, from approximately 6.2 to 7.1 years (Deloitte Centre for Health Solutions, 2023). The average clinical trial cycle is longest for cancer drugs, at more than 11 years, and shortest for infectious diseases, at 4.3 years (Deloitte Centre for Health Solutions, 2023). Although pharmaceutical companies do invest in their own R&D, industry also relies on federally funded discovery research as starting points for asset development—underscoring the need for robust public funding for the U.S. biomedical research enterprise.

Philanthropic gifts are a small but growing aspect of the U.S. biomedical research enterprise's funding portfolio. According to one report, although federal funding for university research grew less than 1% annually between 2005 and 2010, science philanthropy grew and has continued to grow at 5% annually (Murray, 2013).

Philanthropic investments and gifts—when compared to public or private funding—can come with fewer or different restrictions on how the donations are spent. Philanthropic dollars from grateful patients often go to individual researchers rather than their institution, providing individuals with more leeway on what projects they would like to focus on, but providing little benefit to the institution writ large—until the individual researcher achieves a breakthrough product or discovery, which is not guaranteed to happen. Larger gifts and endowments, however, can provide more flexibility and allow institutions and individual researchers to support early-stage research that much federal funding cannot. Philanthropy can be an important source of funding for research focused on innovation and discovery and of support for early-career researchers as they launch their careers (Conn et al., 2023).

Due to venture capital and industry's focus on returns on investment and philanthropy's often narrow and personalized guardrails, many promising biomedical discoveries languish due to lack of funding until their utility is appreciated, which may not happen for years, decades, or ever. The agendas that accompany funding type are preventing the U.S. biomedical research enterprise from producing maximum returns on investment, because products that spent years in development may sit unused until they are translated into diagnostics or treatments by someone willing to risk the time and money on them.

OVERCOMING THE FUNDING VALLEY OF DEATH

Not all ideas can be translated successfully, and even promising discoveries are not guaranteed a path to the patient. To move promising theories into actionable therapeutics, researchers must find funding from venture capital, angel investors, or private equity, or cobble together available government grants to continue their work. Many efforts to find funding fail. This translational support gap is called the "funding valley of death" and prevents the advancement of potential breakthrough therapies from idea to action.

One area of great success in the translation of basic research into marketable therapies was the passage of the 1983 Orphan Drug Act (Swann, 2018). The Act provided financial incentives for companies to pursue drug approvals for rare diseases—conditions affecting so few people that the typical financial calculus precluded industry investment. In the 20 years after its passing, the Orphan Drug Act led to 232 new drug approvals that helped about 11 million patients (Swann, 2018).

Other programs and efforts are attempting to address the funding valley of death, including:

- The Small Business Innovation Research program, which promotes innovation and entrepreneurship and increases private-sector commercialization of publicly funded research discoveries (SBIR STTR, n.d.);
- The Small Business Technology Transfer program, which aims to foster technology transfer between small businesses and research institutions (SBIR STTR, n.d.);
- The Biomedical Advanced Research and Development Authority, which establishes public–private partnerships to bridge translational gaps and has supported the U.S. Food and Drug Administration (FDA) approval of 89 vaccines, drugs, therapies, and diagnostic tools for public health emergencies (medicalcountermeasures.gov, 2024);
- NIH's Clinical Translational Science Awards program, which enhances training in translational sciences and provides academic scientists and small companies with hard-to-access and expensive technologies via direct expert contract support (NIH NCATS, n.d.);
- The Advanced Research Projects Agency for Health, which supports transformative biomedical and health research ranging from molecular to societal innovations for health solutions (ARPA-H, n.d.);
- Efforts from NIH to leverage philanthropic and industry resources for translational discovery by establishing successful public–private partnerships

through the Foundation for the National Institutes of Health (FNIH, n.d.); and
- Efforts from NIH to facilitate clinical trials for meritorious early and mid-stage projects by establishing standing clinical trial networks that help advance early-stage research to proof-of-concept. At that point, industry could pick up and carry projects to approval—if that does not happen, NIH itself undertakes the task of carrying the trials forward (NIH SEED, n.d.).

Even with these programs in place, additional opportunities for facilitating the translation of discoveries into tangible patient benefits exist and should be utilized. The Defense Innovation Unit of the Department of Defense "accelerates the adoption of commercial technology throughout the military," partnering with external entities to "rapidly prototype and field dual-use capabilities that solve operational challenges at speed and scale" (DIU, n.d.). In-Q-Tel, a venture capital firm funded by the Central Intelligence Agency, explores, identifies, and funds emerging technologies and startups that can benefit the U.S. government (IQT, n.d.). The Department of Energy Loan Programs Office "provides attractive debt financial for high-impact, large-scale energy infrastructure projects," helped launch the Tesla Model S, and supported the upgrade of Ford manufacturing facilities to build vehicles with improved fuel efficiency (energy.gov, 2023). Sustained investment in basic, translational, clinical, and manufacturing R&D by all participants in the ecosystem—even when policies and market conditions are adequate to support at-risk investments—will help facilitate translation and more effectively deliver discoveries to market.

COORDINATED AND FOCUSED FUNDING IS NECESSARY TO ADDRESS AMERICA'S HEALTH CHALLENGES

The fragmented and disparate economic models that undergird the U.S. biomedical research enterprise are not producing sufficient investment to develop treatments for several key public health needs. R&D into antimicrobial resistance, for example, is severely underfunded and leaves the American people vulnerable to persistent infections because market realities have forced companies doing this work to exit the field (Bayer Global, 2023). Another area of need is the renewed production of older drugs that have gone through the entire translational process and are now being sold as generics but are in short supply or no longer produced (Noguchi, 2023b). An exclusive focus on profit undervalues the critical nature of generic drugs, which compose 90% of prescriptions in the United States, and ignoring these shortages may leave

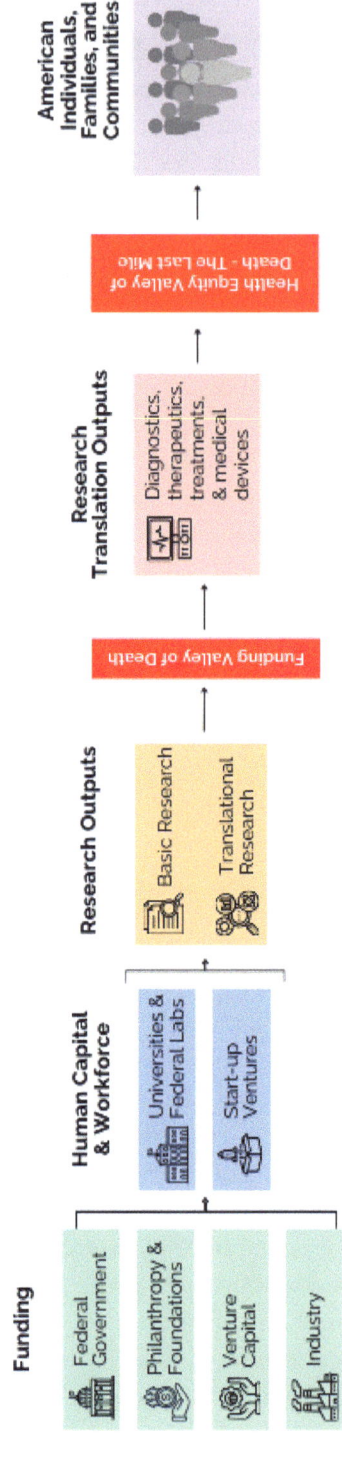

FIGURE 3-3 | Current state of the U.S. biomedical research enterprise.

people who depend on these drugs without access to their more affordable versions (Noguchi, 2023b).

The current U.S. biomedical research enterprise, illustrated in Figure 3-3, despite a wealth of breakthroughs and positive inputs, falls short of its immense potential. The siloed nature of funding sources, as well as their competing agendas, is concerning for the future of the emerging, complex health conditions that threaten American well-being.

The United States needs to break down these silos and develop an overarching vision for biomedical research funding, much in the same vein as the national strategic vision. Although the United States spends more on biomedical R&D than any other nation, federal investment is fragmented across agencies, institutes, and centers, with little cohesion or overarching strategy to address population needs or the social determinants of health. Research expenditures across sectors are driven not by a national mission to improve health, but by motivations such as marketability and profit margins that do not always benefit patients.

CALL TO ACTION

Bringing together federal funders, venture capital, industry, and philanthropy to form a proactive funding body and mechanism will enable the pooling of resources to collaboratively address national biomedical research priorities. The COVID-19 pandemic illustrated the success and power of such partnerships, which should be leveraged more strategically for long-term progress and not only in times of crisis. This funding body should use all available models and best practices to inform its composition and work, but should especially investigate the successes and mechanisms of the Foundation for the National Institutes of Health Accelerating Medicines Partnership and the Advanced Research Projects Agency for Health Investor Catalyst Hub.

The U.S. government is the largest single investor in biomedical research and should take the lead in bringing other investors to the table to co-fund research that addresses the nation's health priorities. The priorities established in the national strategic vision (see Chapter 2) will help direct investment, clearly identify and minimize investment risks, and bring returns on investment in the long term. To better realize the potential of basic science, the funding valley of death that prevents worthy discoveries from being translated into therapeutics and products must also be addressed and eliminated.

Establishing a national strategic vision for coordinated biomedical and health research to improve the lives of Americans will catalyze funders to invest in a focused and synergistic manner. With the federal government bringing venture capital, industry, and philanthropy to the table, their pooled resources could be leveraged to tackle the most serious diseases facing the American people. Relying solely on the government to improve population health is short sighted—much greater gains can be achieved with pooled resources and a shared strategy, and improving the health of all Americans will benefit all Americans.

To realize this vision, the authors of this Special Publication propose the following:

Priority 2-1: A federally established national biomedical research funding collaborative, guided by best practices from existing international models, and federal determinations of how best to organize and allocate shared investments from the government, private sector, and philanthropy. The funding collaborative could be empowered to:
- Analyze successful existing models to develop best practices for the implementation of new methods for financing and accelerating biomedical research;
- Create a large-scale funding model to address the health challenges identified in the national strategic vision; and
- Develop new philanthropic collectives to encourage pooled, strategic gifts that can make a large impact.

Priority 2-2: Federally developed initiatives and funding strategies to specifically address the issue of the "funding valley of death" to translate promising basic research into breakthrough therapies, diagnostics, and treatments—helping to ensure that the full value of the U.S. biomedical research enterprise reaches all patients equitably.

4
A RENEWED FOCUS ON HEALTH EQUITY

The vision of the U.S. biomedical research enterprise at its inception was to improve health for all Americans—it has not yet achieved that goal. Despite massive breakthroughs in chronic diseases such as cancer, cardiovascular disease, and HIV/AIDS, these and other diseases still impact some populations more severely than others. Racial and ethnic minority groups in the United States, specifically, experience worse outcomes in almost every measure of health and wellness compared to their White counterparts (CDC, 2023). The authors of this Special Publication argue that the U.S. biomedical research enterprise has downplayed the importance of health equity for too long, and it is now time for health equity to be centered in U.S. biomedical research, the workforce that conducts this research, and the enterprise itself.

NOT EVERYONE IS RECEIVING THE BENEFITS OF THE U.S. BIOMEDICAL RESEARCH ENTERPRISE

This section of the Special Publication mirrors the successes outlined in Chapter 2 but highlights existing and growing disparities despite hard-earned advances. This close examination of individual outcomes should help to illuminate the dire need for a comprehensive and sustained focus on advancing health equity in biomedical research.

Disparities in Cancer

Despite many successes in reducing cancer mortality in the past 20 years, an in-depth look reveals a more nuanced reality. When age-adjusted per 100,000 people and disaggregated by race and ethnicity, the groups experiencing the highest rates of new cancer diagnoses in 2017–2021 were non-Hispanic

White, non-Hispanic Black, and non-Hispanic American Indian or Alaska Native, in descending order from highest rates to lowest rates (NIH NCI, n.d.c). However, during the same period, the groups experiencing the highest death rates due to cancer were non-Hispanic Black, non-Hispanic American Indian or Alaska Native, and non-Hispanic White individuals, also in descending order from highest rates to lowest rates (NIH NCI, n.d.c). "For all cancers combined, non-Hispanic Black men have the highest rate of new cancer diagnoses" and experience the highest death rates due to cancer of any racial group (NIH NCI, n.d.c). The prevalence of prostate cancer among non-Hispanic Black men is particularly stark (see Figure 4-1).

"For all cancers combined, non-Hispanic White women have the highest rate of new cancer diagnoses" but non-Hispanic Black women have the highest mortality rate for all cancers combined (NIH NCI, n.d.c). Mortality due to breast cancer has generally decreased, but Black women experience significantly higher mortality rates due to breast cancer than any other group (see Figure 4-2).

Today, 72 National Cancer Institute (NCI)-designated centers across the United States perform cancer research and conduct clinical trials to test new treatments and train the next generation of researchers and clinicians (NIH NCI, 2024).

Disparities in Cardiovascular Health

Despite an overall decrease in cardiovascular disease mortality in the past few decades, disparities have increased. One analysis of cardiovascular mortality between 1967 and 2013 finds that although Black individuals experienced 12% higher mortality due to cardiovascular disease than White individuals in 1969, by 2007 the gap had widened to 38% (Singh et al., 2015). Between 1969 and 2011, mortality rates from cardiovascular disease declined for all groups, but mortality decreased most rapidly among the most affluent individuals (Singh et al., 2015). Individuals from lower socioeconomic strata also experienced higher mortality rates than their peers (Singh et al., 2015). Another analysis revealed that people with low education attainment and low income had a higher risk of cardiovascular disease mortality than those with high education attainment and high income (Khan et al., 2024).

After 2012, increases in heart failure mortality have reversed the downward trend in cardiovascular disease–related mortality by 103%, with the greatest reversals seen in people younger than age 45, people aged 45–64, men, non-Hispanic Black individuals, people living in rural areas, people living in the Southern United States, and people living in the Midwestern United States (Sayed et al., 2024).

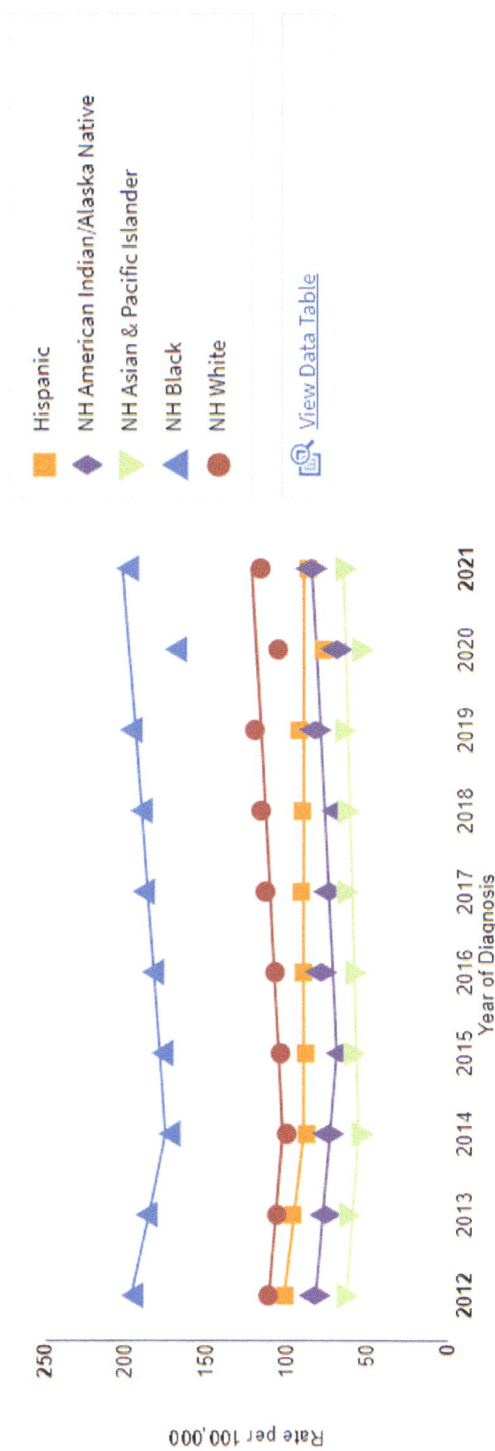

FIGURE 4-1 Prostate cancer: Age-adjusted rate of new cases per 10,000 men by race/ethnicity.
SOURCE: NIH NCI, n.d.c.

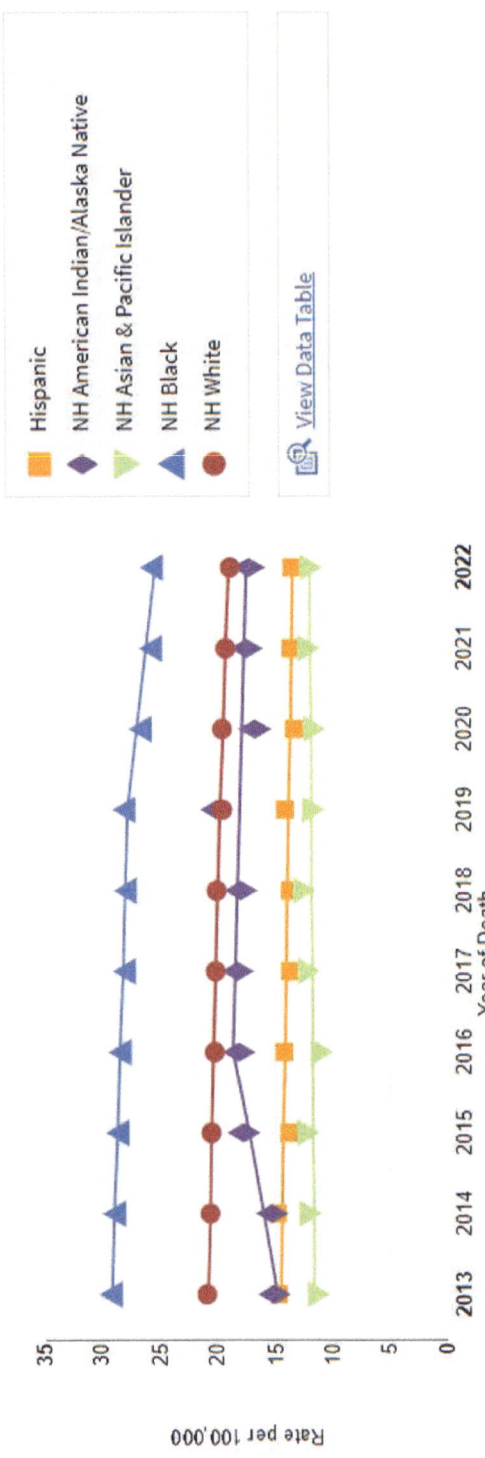

FIGURE 4-2 | Female breast cancer: Age-adjusted death rate per 100,000 women by race/ethnicity.
SOURCE: NIH NCI, n.d.c.

Disparities in HIV/AIDS

Today, more than half of U.S. individuals living with HIV are older than age 50 (HIV.gov, 2023a). Most individuals in this cohort were likely infected when they were younger and have survived to this age because only one in six HIV diagnoses in 2021 were in individuals older than age 50 (HIV.gov, 2023a). Despite a marked reduction in overall incidence and mortality since 1995 due to the availability and use of antiretroviral drugs, between 2009 and 2018, new HIV diagnoses increased in people aged 25–34 and Hispanic men who have sex with men (NIH, 2021). In 2018, 52% of new cases occurred in the American South, where only 37% of Americans reside (see Figure 4-3). In 2021, Black individuals accounted for 40% of new HIV diagnoses in people aged 13 or older, but Black individuals in this age range compose only 12% of the U.S. population (HIV.gov, 2023b). In the same year, Hispanic/Latino patients accounted for 25% of people with HIV but compose only 18% of the U.S. population (HIV.gov, 2023b).

Disparities in Obesity

People of minority race, with lower income, with lower education, and living in certain regions of the United States are at higher risk for obesity than their

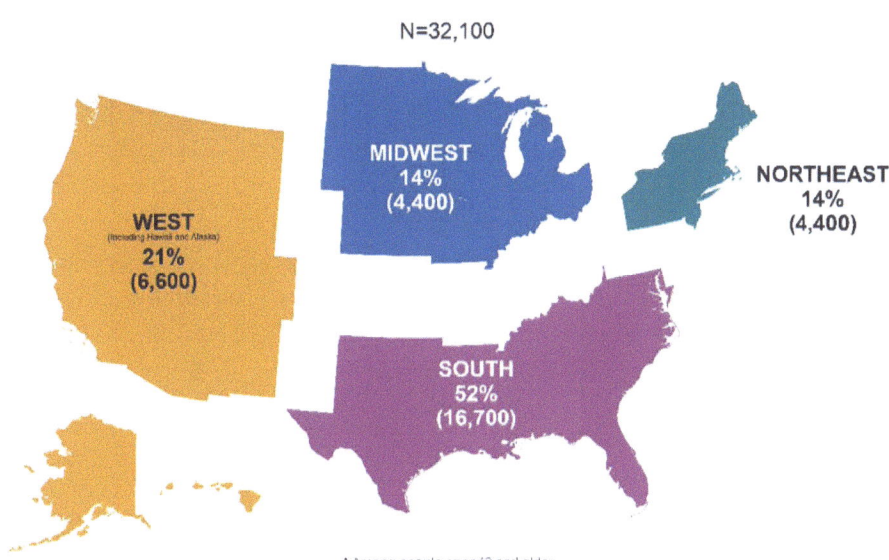

FIGURE 4-3 | Estimated HIV infections in the United States by region, 2021.
NOTE: Among people aged 13 and older.
SOURCE: HIV.gov, 2023c.

peers (Fouad et al., 2022). Black individuals have the highest prevalence of obesity among all groups—49.6%—and Black women have higher rates of obesity than Black men, at 56.9% (Fouad et al., 2022). Geographic disparities are also apparent, as individuals who live in the American South and rural communities are at higher risk for obesity than their peers (Fouad et al., 2022). As mentioned throughout this Special Publication, individuals with obesity are at higher risk for developing diseases such as diabetes, hypertension, and cardiovascular disease, and individuals who experience health disparities related to obesity are also more likely to experience health disparities in these associated conditions, compounding the potential morbidity and mortality from both.

A new class of drugs originally approved for diabetes treatment has begun to be widely used for weight loss. These drugs, six of which have been approved in the United States, can contribute to a 5% to 10% loss in overall body weight (FDA, 2023). However, these drugs are expensive and not always covered by insurance. Even more, prices for these drugs are significantly higher in the United States than in peer nations. An analysis by the Kaiser Family Foundation found that two popular drugs, Ozempic and Wegovy, are five times and four times more expensive in the United States than in Japan and Germany, respectively (Amin et al., 2023). These drugs will likely not be available as more affordable generics for many years, which makes this new intervention effectively inaccessible to many who might benefit from it.

Disparities Among Genders

Individuals who identify as men and women are differentially affected by certain conditions due to factors such as "genetic vulnerabilities to illness, reproductive and hormonal factors, and differences in physiological characteristics" (Vlassoff, 2007). Furthermore, "until recently, a male model of health was used almost exclusively for clinical research, and the findings were generalized to women," effectively excluding women's unique risks from clinical research (Vlassoff, 2007). Women are now increasingly included in clinical research, but still not at parity with men, so disparities across the disease spectrum linger. Some examples of these disparities include:

- Men have a 20% higher incidence of cancer than women, and their death rate is 40% higher. However, disparities vary by type of cancer—for example, "thyroid cancer incidence rates are 3-fold higher in women than in men … despite equivalent death rates … largely reflecting sex differences in the 'epidemic of diagnosis'" (Siegel et al., 2017).

- About 55,000 more women die from stroke each year than men, and stroke is the third highest cause of death for women (AHA, 2023).
- Women are more commonly affected by alcohol- and drug-induced liver disease and show an increased prevalence of acute liver failure (Guy and Peters, 2013). While men tend to misuse alcohol more than women, the relative risk of alcohol-induced cirrhosis in people who consumed 28–41 beverages per week was found to be 7 in men versus 17 in women (Wieland and Everson, 2018).

Health disparities can also compound, existing along both gender and racial/ethnic lines. For example, Black men, compared to all other races, are twice as likely to die from prostate cancer (Lowder et al., 2022). Black women have a higher prevalence of heart disease, stroke, cancer, diabetes, obesity, and maternal mortality than their White counterparts (Chinn et al., 2021).

Black women also have worse cardiovascular health than women of all other groups and experience shorter life expectancy than their White counterparts (Chinn et al., 2021). Black women are three times as likely to die during pregnancy and within 1 year of delivery than their White and Latina counterparts, a disparity that has increased over time (Chinn et al., 2021). Chinn and colleagues note, importantly, "Health outcomes do not occur independent of the social conditions in which they exist," underscoring the need for a comprehensive and sustained approach to health equity within the U.S. biomedical research enterprise (Chinn et al., 2021).

A DIVERSE U.S. BIOMEDICAL RESEARCH ENTERPRISE IS NECESSARY TO PROMOTE HEALTH EQUITY

Data clearly show that diverse teams, especially in science and medicine, lead to improved outcomes for patients, including their "access to care, their perceptions of the care they receive, and their health outcomes, especially for patients of color" (Zephyrin et al., 2023). Beyond directly treating patients, a diverse U.S. biomedical research enterprise workforce is necessary for conducting research to support new initiatives to reduce and ameliorate health disparities and promote health equity. A diverse workforce will help ensure the surfacing of important problems for racial and ethnic minorities that may be otherwise overlooked or ignored by a primarily White workforce; can help build trust in science among the American public; and can help ensure increased participation in clinical trials, thereby generating more detailed data that represents what the American public actually looks like. However, "certain racial/ethnic groups (Black, Hispanic, Native American/Alaska Native, and Native Hawaiian and other Pacific Islander individuals), women, individuals with disabilities, and socioeconomically disadvantaged individuals are persistently underrepresented in the research workforce" (Valantine and Collins, 2015). According to 2021 data, the U.S. biomedical research enterprise workforce is 53.5% White, 26.4% Asian, 9.5% Hispanic or Latino, 6.3% Black or African American, 4.1% unknown, and 0.2% American Indian or Alaska Native (Zippia, 2024). Diversifying the biomedical research enterprise workforce is not only morally right in that it will ensure equal access to jobs in biomedical research for all Americans but will also improve health outcomes for Americans, make research more robust, and advance health equity.

A promising opportunity for diversifying the U.S. biomedical research enterprise workforce pipeline is described in a 2019 National Academies of Sciences, Engineering, and Medicine consensus study titled *Minority Serving Institutions: America's Underutilized Resource for Strengthening the STEM Workforce* (NASEM, 2019b). According to this report, the 700 minority-serving institutions (MSIs) of higher education in the United States enroll nearly 5 million students, which represents about 30% of the U.S. undergraduate population (NASEM, 2019b). Proportionally more undergraduate students are majoring in science, technology, engineering, and mathematics (STEM) fields at 4-year MSIs compared to 4-year non-MSIs (NASEM, 2019b). The report also states that 25% of U.S. STEM undergraduate degrees are conferred by MSIs—a statistic that is not reflected in the data presented above regarding the composition of the biomedical research workforce, suggesting that students graduating from MSIs with STEM degrees are "leaking" from the pipeline between graduation and employment (NASEM, 2019b). The report recommends stronger policies and practices to "intentionally support nontraditional student bodies, particularly those in STEM fields, who may need additional academic, financial, and social support and flexibility given the unique demands and rigor of these fields" (NASEM, 2019b). The high number of American students graduating with STEM degrees from MSIs presents an immediate opportunity to diversify and strengthen the U.S. biomedical research workforce. Readers should refer to Chapter 6 for additional innovative approaches to recruiting and retaining individuals in the biomedical research enterprise, which could include enhanced student loan forgiveness, clearly defined pathways to becoming a principal investigator, and improved postdoctorate positions that include full employment and benefits.

HEALTH EQUITY MUST BE EMBEDDED INTO THE U.S. RESEARCH ENTERPRISE

As the U.S. biomedical research enterprise has been majority White and male for much of its existence, systemic barriers within the enterprise are standing in the way of reducing health disparities and improving health equity. These barriers, outlined below, must be addressed and removed for the enterprise to effectively and appropriately center health equity in its work.

Data Are Not Diverse and Can Be Biased

Researchers have been calculating polygenic risk scores—a predictive likelihood of developing certain diseases—since 2007 (Cross et al., 2022). However, until recently, these scores were based on the original reference genomes used in the Human Genome Project, which came from only 12 donors all located in Buffalo, New York (NIH NHGRI, 2024). In fact, according to NIH, greater than 90% of the participants in genomic studies have been of European ancestry before the publication of the *All of Us* data set in early 2024 (NIH, 2024b). Successful precision medicine requires broad participation across all subpopulations to ensure the availability of data that are representative of every American. These representative data are necessary for generalizing data and applying these data to drug, therapeutic, and diagnostic development, and will hopefully assist in avoiding unforeseen circumstances when a specific subpopulation reacts differently to an intervention because the population at risk was not included in the original research. Progress is being made, but more research is needed to strengthen predictive power for all people. For example, in early February 2024, analyzing the genomes of 250,000 participants, including 50% who were of non-European ancestry, *All of Us* announced the identification of more than 275 million previously unknown genetic variants (NIH, 2024b). These breakthroughs are both critical and long overdue, and diverse data sets must be prioritized moving forward.

Another challenge to comprehensively addressing health equity is the inherent bias in artificial intelligence, now used more and more regularly in health care and biomedical research. Emerging artificial intelligence and machine learning tools are trained on historical data, which could perpetuate existing biases (Manyika et al., 2019). Some examples of bias inherent in training sets include over- or underrepresentation of subpopulations within a data set, bias built into the data set from the scientists who manage it, or an overreliance on single factors such as vocabulary or income (IBM, 2023). Moving forward, tools should be trained on new or real-world patient data to ensure that historic and systemic bias is not perpetuated, and data engineers should be educated on how to ameliorate or eliminate bias in their data sets. Taking too long to address these issues could lead to decreased public trust in artificial intelligence or machine learning tools when public trust in science is already a challenge (see Chapter 2).

One of the largest challenges in identifying and studying health disparities is the need for appropriate and granular data disaggregation because no average patient exists. Likewise, when using racial identifiers as "buckets" for sorting data, disaggregating into ancestral subgroups will likely be the most relevant and accurate way to understand these data, because race/ethnicity is often an assigned label and ancestry captures the genetic origin of one's population (Borrell et al., 2021). Efforts such as the National Commission to Transform Public Health Data Systems, launched by the Robert Wood Johnson Foundation, are only the beginning of the effort to modernize data collection (RWJF, 2021). Federal data collection follows Office of Management and Budget (OMB) definitions, which include only seven categories for race or ethnicity (The White House, 2024). Even so, during the COVID-19 pandemic, many states failed to follow even OMB's minimal requirements, with some mis-aggregating Native Hawaiians and Pacific Islanders with Asian individuals, and some not reporting on Native Hawaiians and Pacific Islanders at all (Kauh, 2021). Although current OMB standards are minimal, agencies need to accurately follow them to ensure a comprehensive understanding of the health of U.S. populations. Further data disaggregation that captures the lived experiences of the entire U.S. population will provide significant insight into misunderstood or misdiagnosed diseases, as well as possible solutions for pernicious health inequities.

A SECOND VALLEY OF DEATH: CLOSING THE LAST MILE

Individuals familiar with the U.S. biomedical research enterprise are likely also familiar with the "funding valley of death" discussed in Chapter 3, or the substantial challenges associated with bringing promising research from concept to market—specifically, procuring funding for this critical but often unprofitable interstitial stage. The authors of this Special Publication believe that a second valley of death, focused on health equity, exists and must be addressed with equal urgency and attention—closing the last mile.

Closing the last mile means getting to people who are hardest to reach, whether due to physical distance or other forms of separation or isolation. The last mile in health care refers to the challenges around providing comprehensive and culturally appropriate health care to marginalized groups; racial and ethnic minorities; Indigenous communities; and people with challenges including disabilities, lack of health insurance, illness, or lack of access to transportation. Many systemic factors contribute to the persistence of the last mile in health care, which further exacerbates health disparities. In addition to being the "farthest from care," individuals impacted by the last mile are also likely those about which the least is known. To achieve health equity in the United States, we must fully research, understand, and mitigate the barriers that sustain the last mile.

In the developing world, the last mile often describes a lack of roads, dirt roads accessible only by foot, and roads that are only seasonally accessible because of flooding or other environmental and climate cycles. In the United States, the last mile in health care likewise separates vulnerable populations from health care services, although by different barriers.

The last mile exists in both rural and urban areas. In rural areas, distance from hospitals that provide specialty care, a lack of local health care facilities or providers, a lack of adequate or any health insurance, and limited or no access to high-speed internet isolate individuals from services. In urban areas, a lack of adequate transportation, crime, or poverty are barriers to accessing health care. Across both urban and rural environments, the last mile exists anywhere individuals experience racism, sexism, or other discrimination that keeps them from seeking care, and is exacerbated by a historical lack of trust in science, health care, and practitioners of both. In addition, people who live in the last mile are typically the most vulnerable members of society, and their circumstances are worsened by a lack of access to adequate health care.

The implications of the last mile are multitudinous but include that 63% of U.S. counties—71% of which are rural—are designated "primary care health professional shortage areas" by the Health Resources and Services Administration (AHRQ, 2023). The digital divide, or the unequal distribution of both technology and technology literacy, impacts rural, low-income, and older individuals most sharply, as "only 55% of U.S. adults over 65 own a smartphone or have home broadband access," only 71% of individuals living below the poverty line own a smartphone, and one in four individuals living in a rural area say that broadband internet access is "a major problem in their community" (Lyles et al., 2022; Read and Wert, 2022). Older and low-income individuals are more likely to have chronic illnesses requiring frequent management than their younger and higher-income peers, and the digital divide can impede their access to virtual care, just as such forms of care are becoming more and more commonplace (Benavidez, 2024; NCOA, 2023).

Despite expanded access to health care through the Affordable Care Act and to Medicaid and Marketplace plans during the COVID-19 pandemic, in 2022, 25.6 million nonelderly American adults did not have health insurance (Tolbert et al., 2023). Of this population, 64% reported that "they were uninsured because the cost of coverage was too high" (Tolbert et al., 2023). A lack of health insurance directly complicates access to preventative and acute health care. Furthermore, when uninsured individuals do seek care, they are more likely to have medical bills or medical debt that they cannot pay, placing them at even greater risk for poorer health outcomes (Tolbert et al., 2023).

In every state where data are available, racial and ethnic minorities are shown to experience disproportionately negative health outcomes compared to their White counterparts, and White individuals are more likely to access preventative care than their racial and ethnic minority peers. More specifically, Black and American Indian or Alaska Native individuals are "much more likely to die" from treatable conditions like diabetes-related complications than their counterparts (Radley et al., 2021). White and Asian individuals are more likely than Black, American Indian or Alaska Native, and Latinx/Hispanic individuals to get an annual flu shot, which greatly reduces their risk of potential complications and mortality due to influenza (Brewer et al., 2021). Last but importantly, although the quality of care varies across states, White individuals generally receive better quality health care than Black, American Indian or Alaska Native, Asian/Native Hawaiian/Pacific Islander, and Latinx/Hispanic individuals (IOM, 2003).

Even when individuals do seek care, discrimination can discourage them from returning for necessary follow-ups, compel them to spend time seeking a new provider, or cause them to avoid obtaining care altogether, all of which can lead to negative health outcomes (Gonzalez et al., 2021). A study by the Robert Wood Johnson Foundation found that Black individuals experience discrimination in health care at three times the rate of White individuals and twice the rate of Latino and Hispanic individuals (Gonzalez et al., 2021). Black women and low-income Black individuals experience even higher rates of discrimination. Given that Black women already experience disparately negative health outcomes, as discussed earlier in this chapter, discrimination that deters or prevents them from seeking or receiving care must be addressed to reduce the disproportionately high rates of morbidity and mortality in this demographic group.

Just as health disparities can and do intersect and exacerbate one another, so can aspects of the last mile. A lack of transportation and a dearth of local health care facilities—aspects of the last mile—can prevent individuals from accessing care. Telehealth and telemedicine services, popularized during COVID-19 and now becoming more and more widely used, appear to be one solution to this problem because individuals can access care from their homes without the need for transportation or to travel hundreds of miles to the nearest hospital (Gelburd, 2023). However, populations that require easier access to care increasingly overlap with those that lack access to high-speed internet or a smartphone, rendering virtual care just as difficult to access as in-person care. One potential solution to this pernicious problem is providing care outside of the hospital or clinic, as many "hospital at home" programs piloted across the country have endeavored to do (Noguchi, 2023a). Additional research is needed to confirm the efficacy and safety of such programs, as well as their ability to scale, but they offer promise for reaching people affected by the last mile.

The authors of this Special Publication have defined the health equity valley of death as such to call attention to this critical, complex, and overlapping set of structural barriers that keep the most vulnerable individuals in the United States from accessing safe, effective, and culturally appropriate care. Sustained attention and research are needed to close the last mile and to ensure, in doing so, that unintended consequences are minimized and the needs of those most impacted by the last mile are centered.

Efforts to address the health equity valley of death will focus on the portion of biomedical research translation that occurs after the funding valley of death. Once a piece of research has been successfully translated into a therapeutic, diagnostic, or medical device, the health equity valley of death obstructs the delivery of these products to people who need them most. Closing the last mile will ensure the effective deployment and delivery of products that were successfully translated from research. The world learned well during the COVID-19 pandemic that an efficacious vaccine does nothing to prevent the spread of disease until it is injected into someone's arm—closing the last mile will ensure that the fruits of the U.S. biomedical research enterprise are available to people who need them—no matter what they look like, where they are located, or how much money they have.

CALL TO ACTION

As the nation reimagines the possibilities of the U.S. biomedical research enterprise, it is critical—and long overdue—to ensure that achieving health equity and reducing health disparities are key goals. To achieve its full potential, the enterprise must be able to share its achievements with all Americans, regardless of race, gender, socioeconomic status, or any other factor. Health inequities are pernicious and complex, but if any enterprise can address them, it should be the U.S. biomedical research enterprise. To achieve this vision, the authors of this Special Publication propose the following:

Priority 3-1: Federal prioritization of research that informs solutions for achieving health equity in the United States, including those focused on the social determinants of health, diversifying the workforce, and the U.S. biomedical research enterprise itself. These research areas could include:

- Increasing trust in medicine, science, and the U.S. biomedical research enterprise itself;
- Mitigating structural and systemic discrimination;
- Delivering care to patients and the communities where they reside, using advances in implementation science to guide these solutions;
- Improving the communication of scientific and medical information; and
- Bolstering community engagement and effective bidirectional dialogue.

Priority 3-2: Federal prioritization of research on the "health equity valley of death"—closing the last mile—to understand and eliminate barriers that are preventing the most vulnerable populations in the United States from receiving and accessing comprehensive, high-quality, culturally appropriate care. Specific research areas could include:
- The digital divide;
- Improving access to health care, specifically for individuals who cannot afford adequate or any insurance coverage;
- Transportation barriers;
- "Health care deserts," or a lack of health care providers—primary and specialty—in a given geographic area;
- Improving trust in science, medicine, and practitioners of both;
- Providing care outside of clinics and hospitals to meet individuals where they are; and
- Reducing racism, sexism, and other discriminatory practices that may keep individuals from seeking care.

5
THE NEED FOR FEDERAL COORDINATION AND USE OF CONVERGENCE SCIENCE

When examining the work, strategy, and outcomes of the federal government, a common observation is that better coordination would reduce redundancies and increase efficiency. Although commonplace, this is a critical observation. Coordinating across federal agencies is a bedrock action for advancing the U.S. biomedical research enterprise. As mentioned in Chapter 2, improved and continuous coordination across federal agencies will both support and be driven by the development of a national strategic vision for the U.S. biomedical enterprise.

The need for federal coordination is so great for two reasons. First, the health challenges faced by America are complex, interdependent, and cannot be solved without collaboration between institutes and centers of the National Institutes of Health (NIH), other agencies of the federal government, and actors beyond. Addressing these challenges requires not only high-level coordination to ensure adequate funding, infrastructure, and person-power but also expertise from many fields of study as scientists, researchers, and clinicians work together to develop new therapies and treatments. The use of convergence science—or "an approach to problem-solving that integrates expertise from life sciences with physical, mathematical, and computational sciences, medicine, and engineering to form comprehensive synthetic frameworks that merge areas of knowledge from multiple fields to address specific challenges"—is no longer a value-add (NRC, 2014). It is required to address the diseases and threats facing the American public today.

Second, current methods for funding biomedical research result in fragmented areas of focus and often produce duplicative or conflicting efforts to achieve the same ends. Better coordination across the federal government—driven by the national strategic vision—will enable all players within the federal government and external agencies to "pull in the same direction." Breaking down silos to facilitate collaboration and movement toward the national strategic vision will not eliminate current efforts or prevent future ones. Rather, the biomedical research enterprise will be better positioned to act more proactively, increase efficiencies and productivity, and make tangible progress toward reversing the health challenges and chronic diseases that currently impact many Americans.

COMPLEX HEALTH CHALLENGES AND PERSISTENT CHRONIC DISEASES

As outlined in Chapter 2, the obesity epidemic is one of the most pernicious, complex, and deadly health trends currently impacting Americans. By some estimates, 50% of the U.S. adult population will be obese by 2030 and 1 in 4 adults will be severely obese—defined by having a body mass index (BMI) greater than 40 (Ward et al., 2019). In addition to its own health impacts, rising rates of obesity and diabetes are likely also contributing to rising rates of mortality from cardiovascular disease (Akil and Ahmad, 2011). Obesity is also known to increase the risk of diabetes, making the two chronic diseases inextricable (Klein et al., 2022). The coupling of progress and reversal in obesity, diabetes, and cardiovascular disease, as well as the known—and unknown—causes of obesity illustrate that efforts to improve human health cannot exist in only one field of science or medicine. Instead, there is an urgent need to coordinate research to uncover the biological, social, economic, geographic, and other underpinnings of disease to enhance education, prevention, diagnostics, and treatments to improve care and treatment for all Americans and reduce existing health disparities.

For example, it is known that obesity and diabetes disproportionately impact minority and low-income populations, with non-Hispanic Black individuals experiencing higher rates of end-stage renal disease than their counterparts, and Hispanic and Asian individuals experiencing higher rates of end-stage renal disease complications (Thornton et al., 2020). To address the complex interplay of disease states as well as the clear health disparities in a manner that prioritizes convergence science, in the future envisioned by this Special Publication, the research agendas set by the National Institute of Diabetes and Digestive and Kidney Diseases; the National Heart, Lung, and Blood Institute; and the National Institute on Minority Health and Health Disparities would be coordinated to appropriately address the interplay between and disparities that arise from the intersection of obesity, diabetes, and cardiovascular disease. Perhaps more importantly, scientists from each institute would intentionally collaborate, share information, and participate in studies together to ensure that the knowledge from each field is brought to bear in real time. Intentional coordination of this type will help address all aspects of a difficult problem and avoid unintended consequences.

In addition to better understanding the molecular underpinnings of obesity, diabetes, and cardiovascular disease and developing drugs and treatments to address these conditions, the United States will need to coordinate behavioral health, mental health, food science, nutrition education, and other experts. This new level of convergence science is required to address these complex health challenges. The authors of this Special Publication believe that the current structure of the U.S. biomedical research enterprise cannot effectively address the obesity epidemic—and similarly complex health challenges—so new and creative approaches and collaborations are required.

Two additional examples of complex problems that require convergence science to solve are existing and emerging infectious diseases and deaths of despair. As the global climate continues to change, animals, insects, and other disease vectors will expand into geographic regions in which they were not previously able to survive, leading to the emergence of new infectious diseases and broader spread of existing infectious diseases. For example, in 2022, the United States reported 2,000 cases of malaria due to travel to areas where malaria is endemic (Mitchell et al., 2024). However, in 2023, at least nine cases were contracted by people who had not traveled outside of the country, meaning that their infectious were locally acquired (Bagcchi, 2023). The World Health Organization classified America as malaria-free in 1970, but these locally acquired cases signal the need to prepare for malaria's potential return (WHO, 2023b). Infectious disease experts, entomologists, climate scientists, civil engineers, and state and local health departments will need to collaborate to adequately prepare for potential increases in malaria and other infectious diseases.

Deaths of despair—or early deaths due to suicide, drug overdose, or alcohol consumption—are another example of a serious and complex health challenge that will require convergence science to address (Beseran et al., 2022). Experts in mental health, addiction science, neurologists, behavioral scientists, and social scientists will need to share information and expertise in new ways to combat these deadly trends. In addition, coordinated federal funding that cuts across agencies and NIH institutes could support real progress toward ameliorating these challenges. Such coordination—of expertise, information, people, and funding—will not only provide a solid foundation for research but also signal that these issues are a national priority.

COORDINATED FUNDING WILL LEAD TO COORDINATED SOLUTIONS

As mentioned in Chapter 2, the national strategic vision will drive coordination in both funding and new approaches to science. Coordinated funding will allow the convergence science necessary to solve these challenging issues to occur—one is not possible without the other.

The current biomedical research enterprise has not evolved to adjust for its own success and growth. Without clear, overarching goals, too many priorities compete for insufficient funds, which results in projects with similar objectives launching in parallel rather than in concert and leads to siloed research focused on only one or two areas of expertise, rather than the broad swath of expertise needed to solve many of the health challenges detailed above and in Chapter 2. Research expenditures across all sectors must be driven by a national mission to improve health, rather than individual agendas or motivations such as profit margins.

THE PROMISE OF PUBLIC–PRIVATE PARTNERSHIPS

Public–private partnerships (PPPs) provide tremendous opportunities to enable and encourage collaboration and convergence science and to accelerate discovery and development to improve human health. These joint ventures should not be reserved for public health crises but should be strategically deployed to advance health and health equity where and when most needed. Three impactful examples are provided below to share best practices and opportunities for how PPPs can help accelerate the use of convergence science across the U.S. biomedical research enterprise.

Foundation for the National Institutes of Health Accelerating Medicines Partnership®

Launched in 2014 by the Foundation for the National Institutes of Health (FNIH), the Accelerating Medicines Partnership (AMP) aims to "improve understanding of disease pathways, facilitate better selection of targets for treatment and identify platforms and processes to accelerate new and effective therapies to patients" (FNIH, 2023a). Every AMP project is a PPP, and AMP currently includes 10 projects, 34 industry partners, 37 nonprofit partners, 16 NIH institutes and cross-institute programs, the U.S. Food and Drug Administration (FDA), and $834 million in funding (FNIH, 2023a). The AMP concept emerged from a meeting with leaders of major pharmaceutical company research and development (R&D) branches who were collectively concerned with lagging productivity in drug development pipelines (FNIH, 2023a). Coalescing around a shared interest in accelerating timelines, reducing costs, and increasing success rates of new therapies, AMP supports PPPs that focus on the rapid development of basic tools that benefit all investors as well as the public and private sectors (FNIH, 2023a). AMP projects include:

- Identifying new, clinically relevant therapeutic targets for Alzheimer's disease and improving validation of identified targets and biomarkers (FNIH, 2023b);
- Developing gene therapies for rare genetic diseases that otherwise would not have commercially viable treatments (FNIH, 2023c);
- Using new data and artificial intelligence to better define the symptoms and characteristics of heart failure with preserved ejection fraction—or diastolic heart failure—which occurs when the left side of the heart cannot fill or pump properly (FNIH, 2023d); and
- Validating biomarkers to better understand the early stages of schizophrenia and predict its progression into psychosis and other outcomes (FNIH, 2023e).

One of AMP's completed projects, Phase 1 of the AMP Lupus Network, has established a nationwide network of clinical sites; optimized high-throughput protocols; and amassed a large sum of data from the analysis of renal tissue, urine, and blood from patients with lupus nephritis (LN) (FNIH, 2023f; NIH NIAMSD, 2024a). LN affects up to 40% of people with systemic lupus erythematosus and often results in end-stage renal disease and death—especially among individuals from racial and ethnic minorities (Pryor et al., 2021). Upon completion of the Phase 1 project, researchers are now beginning to identify biomarkers for LN. The newly established network of clinical sites and protocols will assist in learning more about how the kidneys change as LN progresses, providing a clearer understanding of how patients respond to treatments. The Phase 1 project was such a success that it has been expanded into a follow-up program for the Autoimmune and Immune-Mediated Diseases branch of AMP (NIH NIAMSD, 2024b).

Global Health Innovative Technology Fund

Japan's Global Health Innovative Technology Fund (GHIT) is the first PPP of its kind in Japan (GHP and IFPMA, 2024). GHIT's partners include the government of Japan, the Bill & Melinda Gates Foundation, the Wellcome Trust, and assorted global life sciences companies (GHP and IFPMA, 2024). GHIT invests and manages an R&D portfolio aimed at addressing neglected diseases such as malaria, tuberculosis, and other tropical diseases that afflict the world's underserved populations (GHP and IFPMA, 2024).

To date, the GHIT Fund has invested approximately ¥29.1 billion ($202 million USD) in 118 projects (GHIT Fund, 2023). Fifty-three projects are under way, including "26 targeted and exploratory research projects, 15 non-clinical trials and 12 clinical trials" (GHIT Fund, 2023). Demonstrating the GHIT Fund's partnership strength, "170 partners (59 domestic and 111 global groups) have participated in product development thus far, and the number of Japanese institutions and partnering global institutions has increased dramatically over the past 10 years" as of May 25, 2023 (GHIT Fund, 2023).

The GHIT Fund requires that products resulting from research it funds be appropriate, effective, affordable, and accessible to all, regardless of socioeconomic status. In fact, all grant investment proposals must prioritize open innovation and guarantee that products will be developed on a "no gain, no loss" basis (Slingsby and Kurokawa, 2013); that is, in low-income countries, these drugs will be licensed without royalties, but in middle- or high-income countries, they will be licensed at cost (Slingsby and Kurokawa, 2013).

Operation Warp Speed

The U.S. government launched the PPP Operation Warp Speed (OWS) in May 2020 with $18 billion in federal funding to accelerate the development, manufacturing, and distribution of COVID-19 vaccines (GAO, 2021; Tozzi et al., 2020). OWS involved agencies within the Department of Health and Human Services—the Centers for Disease Control and Prevention, FDA, NIH, and the Biomedical Advanced Research and Development Authority—the Department of Defense, the Department of Agriculture, the Department of Energy, and the Department of Veterans Affairs (NIHB, 2020). The primary function of OWS was to provide private companies, which sometimes partnered with federal agencies or scientists, with funding to develop vaccines and treatments. Several companies received funding—Moderna and Pfizer/BioNTech on an mRNA platform; Janssen and AstraZeneca on a replication-defective, live-vector platform; and Sanofi/GlaxoSmithKline and Novavax on a recombinant-subunit-adjuvanted protein platform (GAO, 2021).

OWS's public financing was critical in developing these desperately needed vaccines, as the federal government took on the financial risk for their development, enabling the private companies to focus not on market profitability but on high-volume production. An article from 2023 said, of OWS, "[i]t's a case study in how the U.S. government can solve complex, urgent problems, and it challenges the narrative that public institutions have lost their ability to dream big and move fast" (Hamel and Zanini, 2023).

CALL TO ACTION

The U.S. biomedical research enterprise has produced an overwhelming number of scientific advances and discoveries since its inception. However, the needs of the American people and the health challenges facing them have changed, and the enterprise needs to change as well. The health challenges causing the most mortality and morbidity among the American public are increasingly complex and varied, and cannot be disconnected from pervasive and deadly health inequities and impacts of the social determinants of health. Initiatives to address these challenges require coordination at both the macro and micro levels.

At a macro level, increased coordination among the federal government and specifically the agencies responsible for biomedical research—notably, institutes of the NIH—is vital. Increased coordination will help eliminate siloed approaches to complex health problems, which divide pools of funding and necessary expertise, putting research projects at an immediate disadvantage. It will also produce funding and workforce efficiencies, remove barriers, and hopefully lead to a new series of breakthroughs to improve the health of the American people.

At a micro level, convergence science is no longer a bonus—it is required to solve 21st-century health problems. The health issues outlined to date in this Special Publication—notably, the complex interplay between obesity, diabetes, and cardiovascular disease—by their very nature require a transdisciplinary understanding and approach to solve. Addressing only the biological aspect of any disease is no longer sufficient to appropriately reduce or eradicate it—expertise from other scientific fields, especially behavioral and social sciences, will be imperative to improving health in the long term. Coordination among federal agencies will support the need for convergence science, and both are necessary to achieve the full possibility of the U.S. biomedical research enterprise.

To achieve this vision, the authors of this Special Publication propose the following:

Priority 4-1: Federal requirement and facilitation of necessary and essential coordination across government agencies, especially the National Institutes of Health and the National Science Foundation, as well as external parties, to enable the use of convergence science,

coordinate funding and strategy, adequately address the increasingly complex and interconnected health challenges facing the nation, and promote information sharing.

Priority 4-2: Federal promotion and use of convergence science in all appropriate projects receiving federal funding.

6
A 21ST-CENTURY WORKFORCE FOR THE U.S. BIOMEDICAL RESEARCH ENTERPRISE OF THE FUTURE

The U.S. biomedical research enterprise would not exist without its strong knowledge capital, uniquely skilled workforce, and pipeline of new scientists. Overall, growth of the U.S. biomedical research workforce has increased over the past few decades, but at a slower rate than peer nations. For example, South Korea's research workforce is growing five times faster than America's, and the European Union and the United Kingdom are also outpacing the United States (OECD, n.d.a). Health profession trainees pursuing postdoctoral training, including physician-scientists in clinical research training, have not increased for more than a decade (see Figure 6-1, orange line labeled "postdocs") (NSF NCSES, 2022a). In the biological sciences in 2020, there were more than four PhD candidates for every one PhD recipient pursuing academic postdoctoral research training (NSF NCSES, 2022a). Between 1975 and 2020, the number of graduate students grew by 51%, while the number of postdoctoral scholars grew by only 27%, indicating that PhD graduates are pursuing careers outside of academia (NSF NCSES, 2022a).

The U.S. biomedical research enterprise cannot reach its full potential without a complement of dedicated and talented scientists currently working and a robust pool of students and trainees interested in making biomedical research their career. Unfortunately, the enterprise is not living up to either of these ideals, and new and innovative approaches to recruitment and retention are necessary to support this new vision for the U.S. biomedical research enterprise.

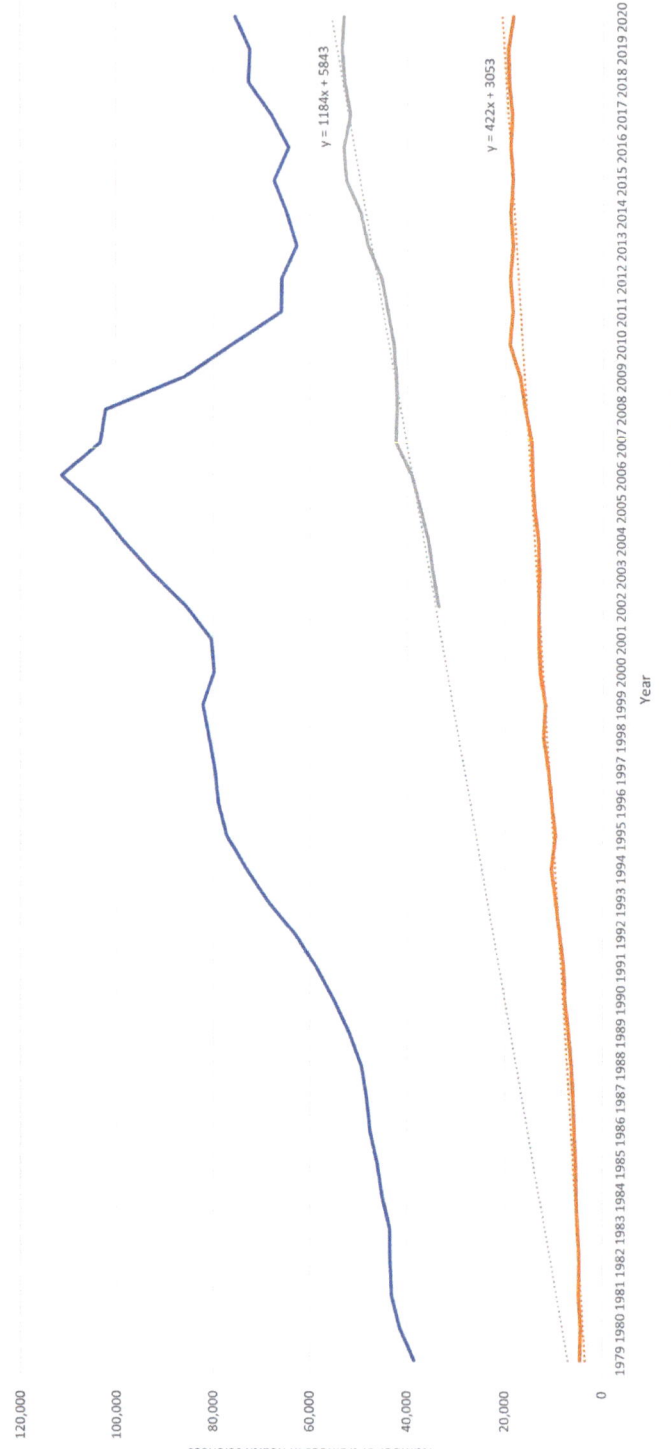

FIGURE 6-1 | Number of U.S. trainees by career stage, 1979–2019.
DATA SOURCES: AAMC, 2021; Yamaner, 2022.

THE CURRENT STATE OF THE
U.S. BIOMEDICAL RESEARCH ENTERPRISE WORKFORCE

The on-ramp to a career in biomedical research is lengthy—beginning with K–12 science, technology, engineering, and mathematics (STEM) education, followed by undergraduate college, proceeding to one or two advanced degrees, and then moving to postdoctoral scholarship and training before full-time employment in academia, the federal government, or industry. This unique compact between postdoctoral scholars and academia originated in the 1870s as an apprenticeship model first adopted by Johns Hopkins University, where PhD graduates take on temporary mentored research experiences to prepare them for independent academic research positions, and has persisted as the default throughout the life of the U.S. biomedical research enterprise (NAS et al., 2000).

Data from 2019 to 2021 show that biological and biomedical science are the only surveyed fields in which the proportion of newly minted PhDs pursuing postdoctoral training decreased (NSF NCSES, 2021). The number of doctorate recipients in the biological and biomedical sciences committing to an industry position after earning their degree has increased to approximately 68% in 2022, compared to approximately 39% in 2002 (NSF NCSES, 2022b). In 2022, approximately 20% of new doctorate recipients in biological and biomedical sciences had committed to academic employment, down from more than 40% in 2002 (NSF NCSES, 2022b).

The same data set also reveals that postdoctoral salaries are lower than those offered by industry or other academic positions across all fields, a strong disincentive for entering postdoctoral training (see Figures 6-2 and 6-3). Median annual salaries for biological and biomedical science doctorate recipients were approximately $52,000 for a postdoctoral position, $68,000 for an academic position, and $110,000 for an industry position (NSF NCSES, 2022b).

Postdoctoral scholars' employment status—whether they are considered employees or trainees—depends on their funding source and determines the benefits they receive (NPA, 2019). Postdoctoral scholars earn historically lower stipends with minimal benefits compared to employment in academia or industry, as illustrated in Figure 6-3. This lack of comprehensive compensation is considered by some to devalue the critical contributions of postdoctoral scholars to the U.S. biomedical research enterprise and provide significant disincentives to pursuing a career in academic research. This perspective appears to be supported by data showing consistently decreasing commitments of new PhDs to postdoctoral positions—a trend that is weakening the U.S. biomedical research enterprise's pipeline of new researchers.

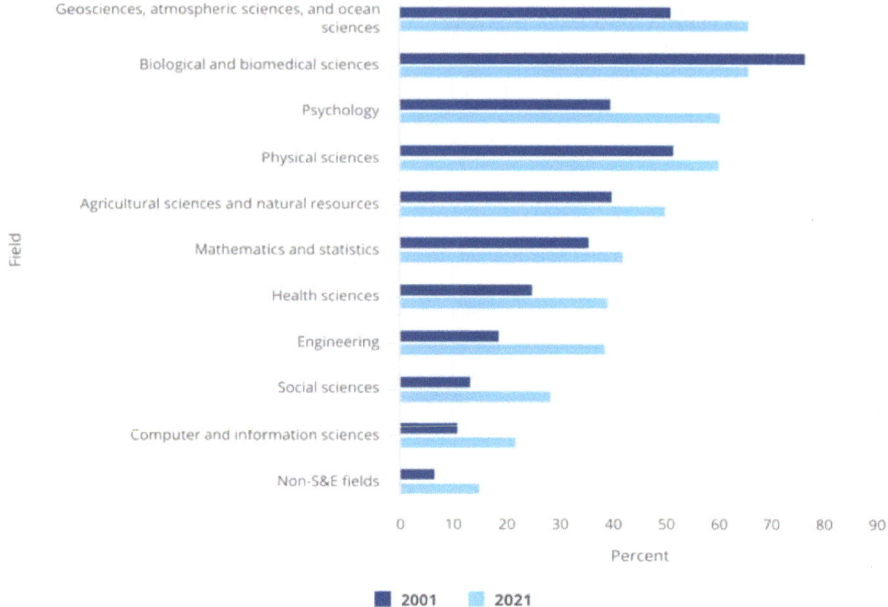

FIGURE 6-2 | U.S. postdoctorate recipients, by broad field, 2001 and 2021.
SOURCE: NSF NCSES, 2021.

CONTRIBUTIONS OF INTERNATIONAL SCIENTISTS

The American education system attracts more than 1 million international students every year, making higher education one of America's top exports, generating more than $44 billion in revenue in 2019 (Khanna, 2021). However, pandemic-era visa restrictions in 2020 reduced new international student enrollment—including K–12 enrollment—by 72% (DHS, 2021).

At the predoctoral level, U.S. citizens continue to represent most of the student population in both health and biological sciences—although the percentage decreased from 87.9% in 1980 to 72.1% in 2020 in science and from 95.1% in 1980 to 89.7% in 2020 in health (NSF NCSES, 2022a). However, at the postdoctoral level, the proportion of international scholars in both fields has exceeded the number of U.S. citizens and permanent residents for the past two decades (NSF NCSES, 2022a). The number of postdoctoral scholars in both health and science professions has been relatively flat for about the past 10 years—growing or declining by less than 10% year over year—signaling a lack of growth in the biomedical research

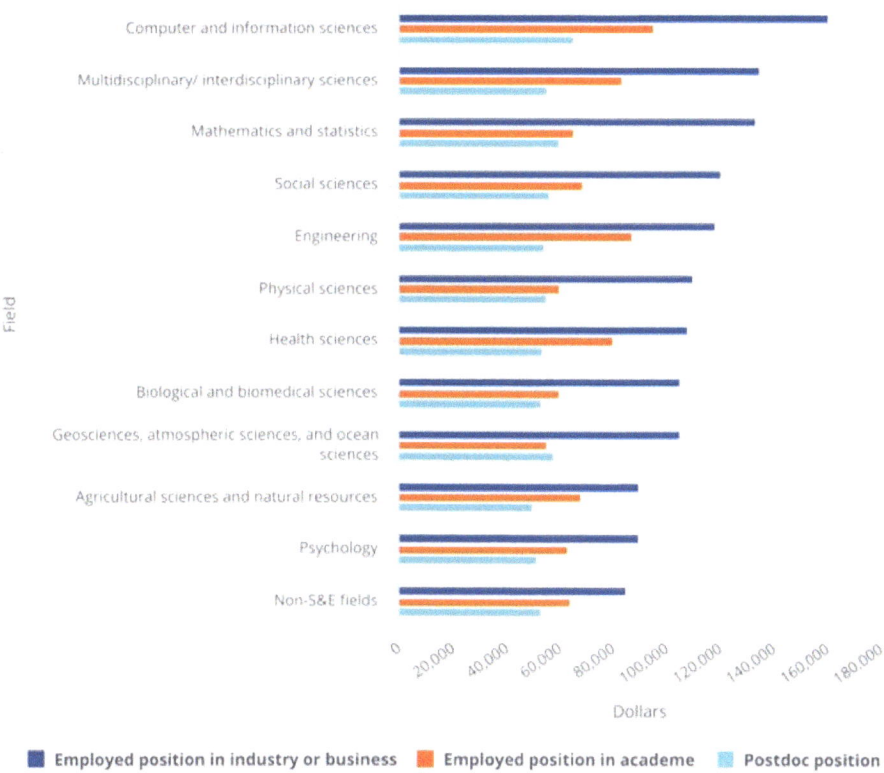

FIGURE 6-3 | Median annual salary of doctorate recipients with definite commitments in the United States, by position type and broad field, 2021.
SOURCE: NSF NCSES, 2021.

workforce (NSF NCSES, 2022a). These shifts are concerning and indicate that U.S. citizens with MDs or PhDs are not pursuing postdoctoral or academic biomedical research training at the rate that foreign-born scholars are.

Compared with 20 years ago, the number of temporary visa holders in health profession training programs pursuing U.S.-based positions after graduation has nearly doubled (NSF NCSES, 2022a). In 2020, 78% of life sciences doctorate recipients had definite commitments to remain in the United States, compared to 72.7% in 2000, demonstrating a strong and growing desire to begin a career in the United States (NSF NCSES, 2020b).

The U.S. biomedical workforce relies heavily on contributions from temporary visa holders as postdoctoral scholars, but the proportion of international predoctoral students has plateaued—and even declined by 10% during the COVID-19 pandemic (NSF NCSES, 2022a). The data show that individuals who come to the United States to earn doctoral degrees tend to stay and accept permanent positions, enriching the research environment and America's knowledge capital. However, temporary visa holders in postdoctoral positions are not eligible to apply for federal funding, limiting the ability of talented individuals to launch independent research careers in the United States. Efforts to ensure the current and future vibrancy of the U.S. biomedical research enterprise workforce should include a focus on reducing barriers to international student participation in U.S. higher education and subsequent transition into postdoctoral scholarship and permanent careers.

COMPETITIVE FUNDING, EMPLOYMENT, AND SALARIES ARE NECESSARY TO ENSURE FUTURE GROWTH

Federal funding for biomedical research has not experienced significant growth since 2003, with overall funding declining between 2010 and 2013 (AAAS, 2022). It is the opinion of the authors of this Special Publication that this static availability of federal research funding has led to a more cautious approach in awards, in that agencies favor what some would deem "safer" projects with longer history and more data supporting their eventual outcomes. This trend also likely favors established investigators over early-career scholars, consequently stifling the launch of promising careers, as well as potentially high-risk, high-reward research proposed by researchers across the career spectrum.

Relatively flat federal funding, compounded with more frequent continuing resolutions in the federal budget process, contributes to instability and uncertainty throughout the U.S. biomedical research enterprise (Lautz and Fano, 2024). This uncertainty is particularly felt by portions of the biomedical research workforce who rely on federal funding. Increasingly frequent threats of government shutdowns—consequently halting research for unpredictable lengths of time—likely make biomedical research less appealing to talented scholars who are already increasingly seeking employment in academia or industry. Congressional appropriations and policies should be mindful of their outsized and immediate impact on the people who make U.S. biomedical research possible. This talent pool sees growing opportunities outside of the federal government and even outside America entirely and cannot be easily replaced once lost.

Many individuals who study biomedical or health sciences in undergraduate and graduate school bring a passion for their work, scientific discovery, and helping others in their everyday lives. However, we, as a nation, cannot continue to rely on their goodwill to carry them from school into postdoctoral positions that are often underpaid—compared to their peer positions—and do not include a living wage or basic benefits such as paid leave and disability coverage. In 2020, the median salary for a male life sciences doctorate recipient with plans to pursue postdoctoral study was $50,000, while the average median salary for the same recipient who planned to pursue full employment was $89,000 (NSF NCSES, 2020a). The math here is clear—for individuals with student loan debt, other debt, caregiving commitments, or who simply want to make a better living—there is no comparison between the compensation of postdoctoral research versus employment. Fellowship and training stipend levels are set annually by the Secretary of the Department of Health and Human Services. In 2024, the highest possible stipend for the most experienced postdoctoral scholar was $74,000—still $15,000 less per year than the median annual salary for someone pursuing full-time employment (NIH NIAID, 2024).

In 2023, the NIH Advisory Committee to the Director Working Group on Re-Envisioning NIH-Supported Postdoctoral Training completed an analysis of the state of postdoctoral training in the United States (NIH Advisory Committee to the Director, 2023). The working group identified "a systemic inertia favoring longstanding, normalized behaviors and incentive structures that do not foster a healthy research and mentoring culture" as a reason why past recommendations to improve the postdoctoral career stage remain unaddressed (NIH Advisory Committee to the Director, 2023). The report also identified fragmentation as a challenge to addressing and correcting systemic problems in workforce development. The NIH Office of the Director responded to this report by raising the pay scales of "predoctoral and postdoctoral scholars at NIH-funded external institutions who are recipients of the Ruth L. Kirschstein National Research Service Awards," but note that "the amended pay levels do not reach the full funding increase recommended by the advisory group" because of existing NIH funding constraints, illustrating that increasing postdoctoral pay cannot be accomplished by a single institution (NIH, 2024c). As a nation, we must acknowledge the critical contributions of our current and future knowledge capital and ensure that its strength persists.

Concerns about the U.S. biomedical research workforce and plans to strengthen the pipeline can no longer ignore the need for adequate and appropriate compensation. Americans cannot ask thousands of current postdoctoral researchers to struggle with their own finances, take unpaid leave, and worry about funding interruptions to help develop therapies, diagnostics, and knowledge that benefit us all.

DIVERSIFYING THE BIOMEDICAL RESEARCH WORKFORCE

In the health professions, the postdoctoral scholar population has become slightly more diverse over time, but the trends are not yet significant enough to signal real progress. Between 2017 and 2021, the number of Black postdoctoral appointees—across all surveyed fields, not just health and biomedical research—grew by 13.1% (Gordon et al., 2023). However, that 13.1% translates to only 133 more Black postdoctoral researchers—from 1,019 in 2017 to 1,1522 in 2021 (Gordon et al., 2023). Black postdocs who are U.S. citizens compose just 26% of all appointees in 2021, a rate that dropped from 29.5% in 2017 (ethnicity and race data were not collected for temporary visa holders) (Gordon et al., 2023). Similar rates hold for Hispanic/Latino postdocs—29.1% growth from 2017 to 2021, from 1,659 to 2,142 (Gordon et al., 2023). Distressingly, appointment rates for American Indian or Alaska Native and Native Hawaiian or Other Pacific Islander postdoctoral researchers dropped precipitously during the same period—negative 36% and 66.1%, respectively (Gordon et al., 2023).

Even more confounding, the increase in Black and Hispanic/Latino postdoctoral scholars has been primarily driven by a decrease in White postdoctoral scholars rather than an absolute increase in underrepresented minorities (Gordon et al., 2023). The necessity for focused recruitment of diverse researchers—particularly American Indian or Alaska Native and Native Hawaiian or other Pacific Islanders—is clear. As described more thoroughly in Chapter 4, a diverse workforce will help ensure progress toward reducing health disparities and achieving health equity, as well as support the U.S. biomedical research enterprise in reaching its full potential.

In terms of gender differences, women in predoctoral health sciences programs in 2020 far exceeded men—76.4% women versus 23.6% men (Gordon et al., 2023). However, the number of male and female postdoctoral appointees in the same health sciences programs is nearly even, at 50.7% women versus 49.3% men (Gordon et al., 2023). It is worth investigating what is happening between graduate school and postdoctoral appointments that is causing the "loss" of greater than 25% of women with advanced degrees. This loss is particularly concerning given that patient–provider concordance can improve patient outcomes and even, in some cases, prevent death (Szabo, 2024). A dearth of female scientists and medical professionals may also exacerbate the lack of attention to health issues that disproportionately impact women.

In science, gender disparities are still apparent but less striking than in the health sciences. The percentage of women in predoctoral science programs was 51.1% in 2020, compared to 48.9% of men (Gordon et al., 2023). When moving to postdoctoral appointments, the gap widens considerably to 41.2% of women compared to 58.8% of men—illustrating a significant gap that demands investigation and intervention (Gordon et al., 2023). Although gender equity is present in the early stages of the biomedical research pipeline, the number of women who leave the field between graduate school and full-time employment is alarming and must be addressed to ensure a diverse U.S. biomedical research enterprise workforce.

THE IMPORTANCE OF PHYSICIAN-SCIENTISTS

Physician-scientists—those "who see patients, teach the next generation of doctors, and do research to understand disease"—are a critical but diminishing section of the U.S. biomedical research enterprise workforce (Utz et al., 2022). Although the exact number of physician-scientists in the United States is difficult to measure, several indicators show that the percentage of physicians who both practice medicine and conduct research is declining (Garrison and Ley, 2022). Physician-scientists receive training that makes them especially well equipped to translate research into treatments and diagnostics, identify rising health challenges, assist in policy negotiations, and communicate science effectively (AAMC, n.d.). However, physician-scientists face the same financial challenges as their peers outlined elsewhere in this chapter, as well as unique challenges including a lack of mentors, reduced basic science education, and the increasing complexity of technology and big data required to conduct research (Utz et al., 2022). The U.S. biomedical research enterprise of the future will be incomplete without the contributions of physician-scientists, and as such, their importance—as well as the unique challenges they face—must be recognized and addressed head-on.

REINFORCING THE PIPELINE ACROSS THE EDUCATION CONTINUUM

The path to entering the U.S. biomedical research enterprise workforce is lengthy, and almost inevitably begins with K–12 STEM education. Exposing young people to careers in science, engineering, technology, mathematics, and medicine is critical to maintaining a robust pipeline of excellent scientists and ensuring that all U.S. children can pursue careers they are passionate about. Many reports, including *Rising Above the Gathering Storm*—mentioned in greater detail in Chapter 1—have called for a renewed focus on improving and expanding K–12 STEM education (NAS et al., 2010). This is not a novel priority area, but it is increasingly critical to maintaining and expanding our robust, effective, and productive U.S. biomedical research enterprise workforce.

CALL TO ACTION

The U.S. biomedical research enterprise cannot achieve its goals without the scientists, health care professionals, researchers, and allied personnel who support its work. Ensuring that the enterprise is a desirable and achievable employment path is critical to ensuring a pipeline of dedicated and intelligent workers who will continue to contribute to the knowledge capital of the United States and the world. However, there are several challenges to achieving this vision, including ensuring that international scientists can continue to come to America, receive an education, and start a career; that salaries and benefits packages for postdoctoral scholars are competitive with comparable positions; that federal funding for biomedical research is more accessible and stable; and that employment in the biomedical research workforce is achievable and welcoming to all—especially Native American or Alaska Native and Native Hawaiian and Other Pacific Islander individuals.

To achieve this vision, the authors of this Special Publication propose the following:

Priority 5: Steps by the federal government and Congress to increase the competitiveness of the U.S. biomedical research enterprise workforce, including the following key priorities:
- Align the U.S. biomedical research enterprise's national strategic vision with the needs of its workforce and set goals to meet those needs;
- Incentivize and implement appropriate, specialized, and necessary education and training for all levels of the U.S. biomedical research workforce—including a reinvigorated focus on K–12 STEM education to reinforce the pipeline at its earliest stages;
- Remove barriers that may prevent full accommodation and integration of international scientists into the U.S. biomedical research enterprise workforce, including expanding eligibility for federal research funding to temporary visa holders;
- Expand Early-Stage Investigator funding opportunities, particularly for physician-scientists, to help stabilize the career-launch phase of becoming an independent investigator;
- Reclassify federally funded postdoctoral scholars as employees and provide full benefits to remove unpredictability and make these positions more attractive, including the following potential approaches:
    o Significantly shortening the duration of postdoctoral training so that scholars gain independence faster,

- Allowing postdoctoral scholars to apply for their own federal funding, and
- Creating PhD-to-faculty positions, which would provide new pathways to stable employment;
• Promote the importance of physician-scientists to the biomedical research enterprise and support their training, education, and professional work, including the following potential approaches:
  - Expanding and increasing scholarships specifically for physician-scientists,
  - Protecting research time and salary support,
  - Connecting postdoctoral scholars with mentors, and
  - Employing innovative and immersive training and research programs; and
• Prioritize and implement innovative approaches to recruiting and retaining the specialized workforce, including by expanding student loan forgiveness, providing new funding modalities for postdoctoral trainees, and creating early career development awards for new investigators seeking to pursue research fields prioritized by the national strategic vision.

7
A RENEWED AND REVITALIZED U.S. BIOMEDICAL RESEARCH ENTERPRISE IS POSSIBLE

The U.S. biomedical research enterprise has advanced science nationally and globally; contributed to increased life expectancy and improved health spans for hundreds of thousands of individuals and their families; and most recently, supported the discovery science underlying, and led the charge in developing and distributing, life-saving vaccines that ended the worst pandemic of the past century. The enterprise supports—directly and indirectly—millions of jobs nationally and globally and welcomes thousands of international scholars to learn, live, and work in America every year. Biomedical research is also a major engine for the U.S. economy, contributing significantly to America's gross domestic product (GDP).

The U.S. biomedical research enterprise has contributed much to the nation and the world in its current state. However, its existing structure, incentives, and modes of operation are quickly becoming barriers keeping the enterprise from reaching its full potential (see Figure 7-1). The future state, efficient operation, and maximum output of the biomedical enterprise are critically important for three main reasons (see Figure 7-2).

Other countries are beginning to contribute significantly more—financially and in terms of workforce—to their own biomedical research enterprises. Although the United States currently contributes the most money toward our enterprise, in terms of overall national GDP, many peer nations are investing proportionally more of their GDPs, signifying an increasing commitment to strengthening their national research efforts. The United States has long been the global leader in scientific innovation, medical breakthroughs, and advancing basic science. Without refocused attention and investment in our biomedical research enterprise, we stand to lose our place of leadership.

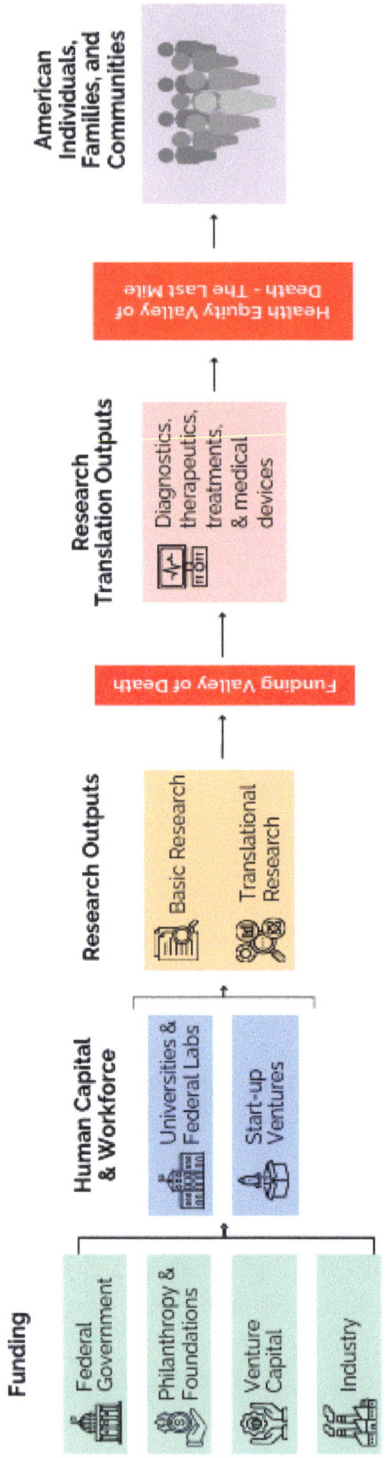

FIGURE 7-1 | Current state of the U.S. biomedical research enterprise.

| 103

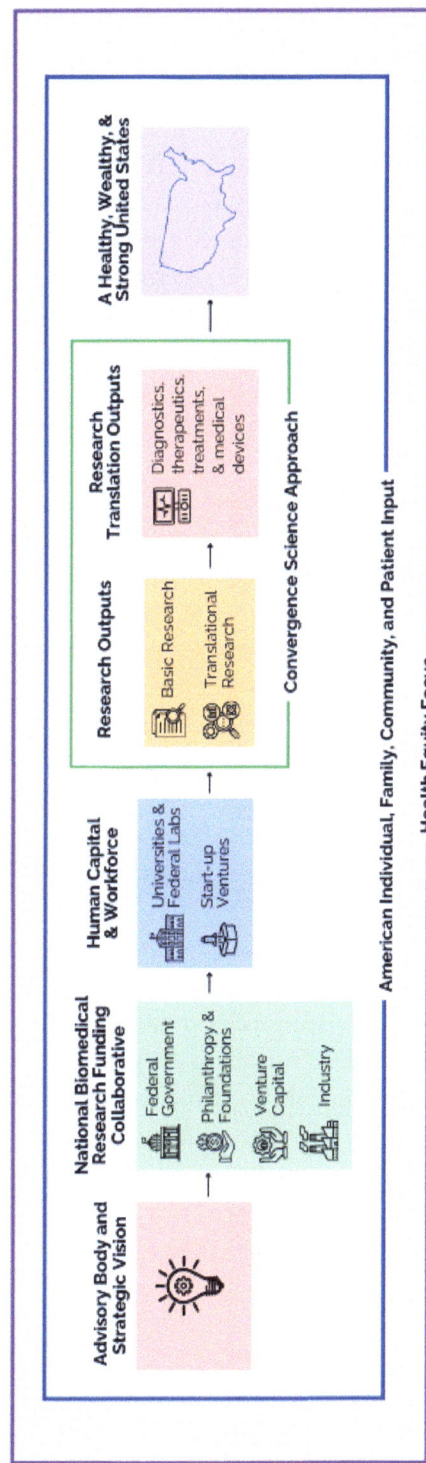

FIGURE 7-2 | Future state of the U.S. biomedical research enterprise.

The most critical and deadly health challenges threatening our nation are complex and interconnected, and will only be solved with convergence science. The U.S. biomedical research enterprise has made great strides in reducing morbidity and mortality for many threats to American health—notably, cancer, cardiovascular disease, and HIV/AIDS. However, the health threats that are currently most damaging and fatal to the American people are increasingly complicated, interconnected with other health issues, and influenced by social determinants of health. Therefore, these threats can only be addressed through collaboration between and among many different fields of biomedical science, social science, and medicine. The U.S. biomedical research enterprise, in its current state, is not positioned to facilitate and encourage convergence science at the scale necessary to make true and lasting headway on improving American health in the long term, and as such, needs to be reimagined and restructured.

A more effective and efficient enterprise will contribute to and grow the U.S. economy. The U.S. biomedical research enterprise spent more than $245 billion on research and development in 2020, a full 3.4% of the total U.S. GDP (Anderson and Moris, 2023; Research!America and Teconomy Partners, LLC, 2022). Despite this massive investment, because of the siloed and fragmented nature of the enterprise, initiatives investigating the same questions are launched in parallel, agendas are dictated by funding rather than need, and projects that could benefit most Americans may not be pursued if they are not profitable. A reimagined system, with a national strategic vision guiding decision making and funding, would contribute more directly to growing the U.S. economy, feed the nation's GDP, and indirectly benefit the economy and GDP by providing more years of healthful life to all Americans.

The authors of this Special Publication believe in the strength, power, and impact of the U.S. biomedical research enterprise to power the economy and improve health for all. The actions laid out in this Special Publication, when taken together, will provide the foundation for the U.S. biomedical research enterprise of the future. As a nation, we have already contributed so much—financially, professionally, and personally—to support and advance the enterprise. We owe it to ourselves—and our children and grandchildren—to ensure that biomedical research, conducted effectively, efficiently, and strategically, benefits all of America.

REFERENCES

No author. 2021. Alzheimer's disease facts and figures. *Alzheimer's & Dementia* 17(3):327–406. https://doi.org/10.1002/alz.12328.

No author. 2022a. Lives saved by COVID-19 vaccines. *Journal of Paediatric and Child Health* 10.1111/jpc.16213. https://doi.org/10.1111/jpc.16213.

No author. 2022b. 2022 Alzheimer's disease facts and figures. *Alzheimer's & Dementia* 18(4):700–789. https://doi.org/10.1002/alz.12638.

Achenbach, J., D. Keating, L. McGinley, A. Johnson, and J. Chikwendiu. 2023. An epidemic of chronic illness is killing us too soon. *The Washington Post*, October 3. Available at: https://www.washingtonpost.com/health/interactive/2023/american-life-expectancy-dropping (accessed May 25, 2024).

Acuña-Villaorduña, A., J. Celebre Baranda, J. Boehmer, L. Fashoyin-Aje, and S. D. Gore. 2023. Equitable access to clinical trials: How do we achieve it? *American Society of Clinical Oncology Educational Book* 43. https://doi.org/10.1200/EDBK_389838.

Advanced Research Projects Agency–Energy (ARPA-E). n.d. *About.* Available at: https://arpa-e.energy.gov/about (accessed May 24, 2024).

Advanced Research Projects Agency for Health (ARPA-H). n.d. *Home.* Available at: https://arpa-h.gov (accessed May 27, 2024).

Agency for Healthcare Research and Quality (AHRQ). 2023. *2023 National Healthcare Quality and Disparities Report.* Available at: https://www.ncbi.nlm.nih.gov/books/NBK600463 (accessed May 27, 2024).

Akil, L., and H. A. Ahmad. 2011. Relationships between obesity and cardiovascular diseases in four southern states and Colorado. *Journal of Health Care for the Poor and Underserved* 22(4 Suppl):61–72. https://doi.org/10.1353/hpu.2011.0166.

American Association for the Advancement of Science (AAAS). 2022. *Historical trends in federal R&D.* Available at: https://www.aaas.org/programs/r-d-budget-and-policy/historical-trends-federal-rd (accessed May 27, 2024).

American Cancer Society (ACS). 2023. American Cancer Society releases latest cancer statistics, launches initiative to address prostate cancer resurgence and disparities. *American Cancer Society*, January 12. Available at: https://pressroom.cancer.org/FactsandFigures23 (accessed May 23, 2024).

American Heart Association (AHA). 2023. *Women and risk of stroke infographic.* Available at: https://www.goredforwomen.org/en/know-your-risk/risk-factors/risk-of-stroke-in-women-infographic (accessed May 27, 2024).

Amin, K., I. Telesford, R. Singh, and C. Cox. 2023. How do prices of drugs for weight loss in the U.S. compare to peer nations' prices? *Peterson-KFF Health System Tracker.* Available at: https://www.healthsystemtracker.org/brief/prices-of-drugs-for-weight-loss-in-the-us-and-peer-nations (accessed May 27, 2024).

Anderson, G., and F. Moris. 2023. Federally funded R&D declines as a share of GDP and total R&D. *NSF NCSES,* June 13. Available at: https://ncses.nsf.gov/pubs/nsf23339 (accessed May 31, 2024).

Antara. 2013. Singapore's Biopolis: A success story. *Antara*, October 17. Available at: https://en.antaranews.com/news/91149/singapores-biopolis-a-success-story (accessed May 26, 2024).

Arias, E., B. Tejada-Vera, K. D. Kochanek, and F. B. Ahmad. 2022. Provisional life expectancy estimates for 2021. *Vital Statistics Rapid Release* 23. https://dx.doi.org/10.15620/cdc:118999.

Association of American Medical Colleges (AAMC). 2021. *2021 fall applicant, matriculant, and enrollment data tables.* Available at: https://www.aamc.org/media/57761/download?attachment (accessed June 20, 2024).

AAMC. n.d. *Physician-scientists.* Available at: https://www.aamc.org/what-we-do/mission-areas/medical-research/physician-scientist (accessed July 3, 2024).

Azoulay, P., D. Li, J. S. Graff Zivin, and B. N. Sampat. 2019. Public R&D investments and private-sector patenting: Evidence from NIH funding rules. *The Review of Economic Studies* 86(1):117–152. https://doi.org/10.1093/restud/rdy034.

Bagcchi, S. 2023. Locally acquired malaria cases in the USA. *The Lancet Infectious Diseases* 23(1):E401. https://doi.org/10.1016/S1473-3099(23)00581-9.

Bayer Global. 2023. New AMR action fund steps in to save collapsing antibiotic pipeline. *Bayer Global*, August 10. Available at: https://www.bayer.com/en/news-stories/new-amr-action-fund-steps-in-to-save-collapsing-antibiotic-pipeline (accessed May 27, 2024).

Beam Therapeutics. 2023. Beam Therapeutics announces first patient dosed in Phase 1/2 trial of BEAM-201 in relapsed, refractory T-ALL/T-LL. *Beam Therapeutics*, September 5. Available at: https://investors.beamtx.com/news-releases/news-release-details/beam-therapeutics-announces-first-patient-dosed-phase-12-trial (accessed May 24, 2024).

Benavidez, G. A., W. E. Zahnd, P. Hung, and J. M. Eberth. 2024. Chronic disease prevalence in the US: Sociodemographic and geographic variations by zip code tabulation area. *Preventing Chronic Disease* 21:230267. http://dx.doi.org/10.5888/pcd21.230267.

Beseran, E., J. M. Pericàs, L. Cash-Gibson, M. Ventura-Cots, K. M. Pollack Porter, and J. Benach. 2022. Deaths of despair: A scoping review on the social determinants of drug overdose, alcohol-related liver disease and suicide. *International Journal of Environmental Research and Public Health* 19(19):12395. https://doi.org/10.3390/ijerph191912395.

Blakeslee, L., Z. Caplan, J. A. Meyer, M. A. Rabe, and A. W. Roberts. 2023. *Age and sex composition: 2020, 2020 Census briefs.* C2020BR-06, May. Available at: https://www2.census.gov/library/publications/decennial/2020/census-briefs/c2020br-06.pdf (accessed July 3, 2024).

Bloom, D. E., A. Khoury, V. Kufenko, and K. Prettner. 2020. *Spurring Economic Growth Through Human Development: Research Results and Guidance for Policymakers.* Program on the Global Demography of Aging at Harvard University Working Paper No. 183. Available at: https://www.hsph.harvard.edu/pgda/wp-content/uploads/sites/1288/2020/02/183_Spurring-economic-growth-through-human-development_feb2020.pdf (accessed May 24, 2024).

BlueCross BlueShield. 2024. *BCBS health index.* Available at: https://www.bcbs.com/the-health-of-america/health-index (accessed May 24, 2024).

Borrell, L. N., J. R. Elhawary, E. Fuentes-Afflick, J. Witonsky, N. Bhakta, A. H. B. Wu, K. Bibbins-Domingo, J. R. Rodríguez-Santana, M. A. Lenoir, J. R. Gavin III, R. A. Kittles, N. A. Zaitlen, D. S. Wilkes, N. R. Powe, E. Ziv, and E. G. Burchard. 2021. Race and genetic ancestry in medicine—A time for reckoning with racism. *The New England Journal of Medicine* 384:474–480. https://doi.org/10.1056/NEJMms2029562.

Braveman, P., J. Acker, E. Arkin, D. Proctor, A. Gillman, K. A. McGeary, and G. Mallya. 2018. *Wealth matters for health equity.* Robert Wood Johnson Foundation, Princeton, NJ. Available at: https://www.rwjf.org/en/insights/our-research/2018/09/wealth-matters-for-health-equity.html (accessed May 24, 2024).

Brewer, L. I., M. J. Ommerborn, A. Le Nguyen, and C. R. Clark. 2021. Structural inequities in seasonal influenza vaccination rates. *BMC Public Health* 21:1166. https://doi.org/10.1186/s12889-021-11179-9.

Brookmeyer, R., S. Gray, and C. Kawas. 2011. Projections of Alzheimer's disease in the United States and the public health impact of delaying disease onset. *American Journal of Public Health* 88(9):1337–1342. https://doi.org/10.2105/AJPH.88.9.1337.

Burke, A., A. Okrent, and K. Hale. 2022. The state of U.S. science and engineering 2022. *NSF NCSES*, January 18. Available at: https://ncses.nsf.gov/pubs/nsb20221/u-s-and-global-research-and-development (accessed May 27, 2024).

Bush, V. 1945. *Science—The endless frontier.* Available at: https://www.nsf.gov/od/lpa/nsf50/vbush1945.htm (accessed May 23, 2024).

Cao, C., R. P. Suttmeier, and D. F. Simon. 2006. China's 15-year science and technology plan. *Physics Today.* Available at: https://china-us.uoregon.edu/pdf/final%20print%20version.pdf (accessed May 26, 2024).

Centers for Disease Control and Prevention (CDC). 2023. *Racism and health.* Available at: https://www.cdc.gov/minorityhealth/racism-disparities/index.html (accessed May 26, 2024).

CDC. 2024a. *National diabetes statistics report.* Available at: https://www.cdc.gov/diabetes/php/data-research/?CDC_AAref_Val=https://www.cdc.gov/diabetes/data/statistics-report/index.html (accessed May 25, 2024).

CDC. 2024b. *Suicide data and statistics.* Available at: https://www.cdc.gov/suicide/facts/data.html?CDC_AAref_Val=https://www.cdc.gov/suicide/suicide-data-statistics.html (accessed May 25, 2024).

CDC. 2024c. *Childhood obesity facts.* Available at: https://www.cdc.gov/obesity/php/data-research/childhood-obesity-facts.html?CDC_AAref_Val=https://www.cdc.gov/obesity/data/childhood.html (accessed May 25, 2024).

CDC. 2024d. *United States cancer statistics: Data visualizations.* Available at: https://gis.cdc.gov/Cancer/USCS/#/Trends (accessed June 19, 2024).

Centers for Disease Control and Prevention, National Center for Health Statistics (CDC NCHS). 2018. *Interactive summary health statistics for adults.* Available at: https://wwwn.cdc.gov/NHISDataQueryTool/SHS_adult/index.html (accessed July 3, 2024).

CDC NCHS. 2024. U.S. overdose deaths decrease in 2023, first time since 2018. *CDC NCHS*, May 15. Available at: https://www.cdc.gov/nchs/pressroom/nchs_press_releases/2024/20240515.htm (accessed May 29, 2024).

Centers for Medicare & Medicaid Services (CMS). 2023. *Historical.* Available at: https://www.cms.gov/data-research/statistics-trends-and-reports/national-health-expenditure-data/historical (accessed May 24, 2024).

Chelak, K., and S. Chakole. 2023. The role of social determinants of health in promoting health equality: A narrative review. *Cureus* 15(1):e33425. https://doi.org/10.7759/cureus.33425.

Cheung, T. M., B. Naughton, and E. Hagt. 2022. China's roadmap to becoming a science, technology, and innovation great power in the 2020s and beyond: Assessing its medium- and long-term strategies and plans. *UC Institute on Global Conflict and Cooperation*, July. Available at: https://ucigcc.org/wp-content/uploads/2022/07/Ocea-revised-19-July-2022-1.pdf (accessed May 26, 2024).

Chinn, J. J., I. K. Martin, and N. Redmond. 2021. Health equity among Black women in the United States. *Journal of Women's Health* 30(2):212–219. https://doi.org/10.1089/jwh.2020.8868.

City of Hope. 2023. What's driving the improvement in U.S. cancer survival rates? *City of Hope*, January 26. Available at: https://www.cancercenter.com/community/blog/2023/01/cancer-survival-rates-are-improving (accessed May 23, 2024).

Coalition for Epidemic Preparedness Innovations (CEPI). 2024. *DISEASE X—What it is, and what it is not*. Available at: https://cepi.net/disease-x-what-it-and-what-it-not (accessed May 25, 2024).

Collins, F. S., and A. S. Fauci. 2010. AIDS in 2010 – How we're living with HIV. *Parade*, May 23. Available at: https://www.nih.gov/sites/default/files/research-training/aids-in-2010-how-were-living-with-hiv.pdf (accessed May 23, 2024).

Congressional Research Service (CRS). 2015. *The America COMPETES Acts: An overview*. Available at: https://www.everycrsreport.com/files/20150727_R43880_933b63e2b44d18b4b2af98acdbef9fbc43822612.pdf (accessed May 24, 2024).

CRS. 2022. *Global research and development expenditures: Fact sheet*. Available at: https://sgp.fas.org/crs/misc/R44283.pdf (accessed May 23, 2024).

Conn, R. W., P. F. Cowhey, J. S. Graff Zivin, and C. L. Martin. 2023. *Science, Philanthropy, and American Leadership*. National Bureau of Economic Research Working Paper 31718. https://doi.org/10.3386/w31718.

Cross, B., R. Turner, and M. Pirmohamed. 2022. Polygenic risk scores: An overview from bench to bedside for personalised medicine. *Frontiers in Genetics* 13:1000667. https://doi.org/10.3389/fgene.2022.1000667.

Curtin, S. C., Tejada-Vera, B., & Bastian, B. A. 2023. Deaths: Leading causes for 2020. *National Vital Statistics Reports* 72(13). Available at: https://www.cdc.gov/nchs/data/nvsr/nvsr72/nvsr72-13.pdf (accessed June 19, 2024).

Deerfield. n.d. *Explore the Deerfield network*. Available at: https://deerfield.com (accessed May 27, 2024).

Defense Innovation Unit (DIU). n.d. *We are building a more secure world*. Available at: https://www.diu.mil/about (accessed May 27, 2024).

Deloitte Centre for Health Solutions. 2023. *Seize the digital momentum: Measuring the return from pharmaceutical innovation 2022.* Available at: https://www2.deloitte.com/content/dam/Deloitte/uk/Documents/life-sciences-healthcare/deloitte-uk-seize-digital-momentum-rd-roi-2022.pdf (accessed May 27, 2024).

Department of Health and Human Services Office of Minority Health (HHS OMH). n.d. *Heart disease and African-Americans.* Available at: https://minorityhealth.hhs.gov/heart-disease-and-african-americans (accessed May 24, 2024).

Department of Homeland Security (DHS). 2021. SEVIS by the numbers: A look at the impact of COVID-19. *DHS*, March 31. Available at: https://studyinthestates.dhs.gov/2021/03/sevis-by-the-numbers-a-look-at-the-impact-of-covid-19 (accessed May 27, 2024).

Diabetes Research Institute Foundation (DRIF). 2023. *Diabetes statistics.* Available at: https://diabetesresearch.org/diabetes-statistics (accessed May 24, 2024).

DukeNUS Medical School. 2022. Duke and NUS reaffirm commitment to Duke-NUS partnership with agreement renewal. *DukeNUS*, October 14. Available at: https://www.duke-nus.edu.sg/allnews/duke-nus-phase-iv-agreement (accessed May 26, 2024).

Embassy of the People's Republic of China in the Hellenic Republic. 2004. *Development of science and technology in China.* Available at: http://gr.china-embassy.gov.cn/eng/kxjs/zgkj/200408/t20040803_3367254.htm (accessed May 26, 2024).

energy.gov. 2023. *History: Loan programs office.* Available at: https://www.energy.gov/lpo/history (accessed May 27, 2024).

Esser, M. B., A. Sherk, Y. Liu, and T. S. Naimi. 2024. Deaths from excessive alcohol use—United States, 2016–2021. *Morbidity and Mortality Weekly Report* 73(8):154–161. http://dx.doi.org/10.15585/mmwr.mm7308a1.

European Commission. 2020. *Research and innovation strategy 2020–2024.* Available at: https://research-and-innovation.ec.europa.eu/strategy/strategy-2020-2024_en (accessed May 26, 2024).

European Commission. 2021a. *Horizon Europe.* Available at: https://research-and-innovation.ec.europa.eu/funding/funding-opportunities/funding-programmes-and-open-calls/horizon-europe_en (accessed May 26, 2024).

European Commission. 2021b. *Horizon Europe: Budget.* Available at: https://op.europa.eu/en/publication-detail/-/publication/1f107d76-acbe-11eb-9767-01aa75ed71a1 (accessed May 26, 2024).

European Commission. 2021c. *Horizon Europe Cluster 1: Health*. Available at: https://research-and-innovation.ec.europa.eu/funding/funding-opportunities/funding-programmes-and-open-calls/horizon-europe/cluster-1-health_en (accessed May 26, 2024).

European Commission. 2023. *Commission staff working document: Evidence framework on monitoring and evaluation of Horizon Europe*. Available at: https://research-and-innovation.ec.europa.eu/document/download/e78eceb1-0859-4192-9117-5bdf4b5cf594_en?filename=swd-2023-132-monitoring-evaluation-he.pdf (accessed May 26, 2024).

European Commission. 2024. Horizon 2020 evaluation shows that investment in EU research and innovation greatly pays off. *European Commission*, January 29. Available at: https://ec.europa.eu/commission/presscorner/detail/en/IP_24_461 (accessed May 26, 2024).

Forsythe, L. P., K. L. Carman, V. Szydlowski, L. Fayish, L. Davidson, D. H. Hickam, C. Hall, G. Bhat, D. Neu, L. Stewart, M. Jalowsky, N. Aronson, and C. U. Anyanwu. 2019. Patient engagement in research: Early findings from the Patient-Centered Outcomes Research Institute. *Health Affairs* 38(3):359367. https://doi.org/10.1377/hlthaff.2018.05067.

Fouad, M. N., K. J. Waugaman, and G. R. Dutton. 2022. The complex contributors to obesity-related health disparities: Introduction to the special issue. *American Journal of Preventive Medicine* 63(1):S1–S5. https://doi.org/10.1016/j.amepre.2022.03.022.

Foundation for the National Institutes of Health (FNIH). 2023a. *Accelerating Medicines Partnership (AMP)*. Available at: https://fnih.org/our-programs/accelerating-medicines-partnership-amp (accessed May 26, 2024).

FNIH. 2023b. *AMP Alzheimer's disease 1.0*. Available at: https://fnih.org/our-programs/accelerating-medicines-partnership-amp/amp-alzheimers-disease-1-0 (accessed May 26, 2024).

FNIH. 2023c. *AMP bespoke gene therapy consortium*. Available at: https://fnih.org/our-programs/accelerating-medicines-partnership-amp/bespoke-gene-therapy-consortium-bgtc (accessed May 26, 2024).

FNIH. 2023d. *AMP heart failure*. Available at: https://fnih.org/our-programs/accelerating-medicines-partnership-amp/amp-heart-failure (accessed May 26, 2024).

FNIH. 2023e. *AMP schizophrenia*. Available at: https://fnih.org/our-programs/accelerating-medicines-partnership-amp/amp-schizophrenia (accessed May 26, 2024).

FNIH. 2023f. *AMP rheumatoid arthritis, systemic lupus erythematosus.* Available at: https://fnih.org/our-programs/accelerating-medicines-partnership-amp/amp-rheumatoid-arthritis-and-lupus (accessed May 26, 2024).

FNIH. n.d. *Building bridges to breakthroughs.* Available at: https://fnih.org (accessed May 27, 2024).

Garnett, M. F., and S. C. Curtin. 2023. Suicide mortality in the United States, 2001–2021. *NCHS Data Brief* 464. https://dx.doi.org/10.15620/cdc:125705.

Garrison, H. H., and T. J. Ley. 2022. Physician-scientists in the United States at 2020: Trends and concerns. *The FASEB Journal.* https://doi.org/10.1096/fj.202200327.

Gelburd, R. 2023. Telehealth utilization grew 7% nationally in January 2023. *American Journal of Managed Care*, April 4. Available at: https://www.ajmc.com/view/contributor-telehealth-utilization-grew-7-nationally-in-january-2023 (accessed July 3, 2024).

Global Health Innovative Technology Fund (GHIT Fund). 2023. Government of Japan expresses its pledge of US$200 million to GHIT Fund/UNDP replenishment. *GHIT Fund*, May 25. Available at: https://www.ghitfund.org/newsroom/press/detail/384/en (accessed May 26, 2024).

Global Health Progress and International Federation of Pharmaceutical Manufacturers and Associations (GHP and IFPMA). 2024. *Global Health Innovative Technology (GHIT) Fund.* Available at: https://globalhealthprogress.org/collaboration/global-health-innovative-technology-ghit-fund (accessed May 26, 2024).

Gonzalez, D., L. Skopec, M. McDaniel, and G. M. Kenney. 2021. *Perceptions of discrimination and unfair judgment while seeking health care: Findings from the September 11–28 coronavirus tracking survey.* Urban Institute and Robert Wood Johnson Foundation. Available at: https://www.rwjf.org/en/insights/our-research/2021/03/perceptions-of-discrimination-and-unfair-judgment-while-seeking-health-care.html (accessed July 3, 2024).

Gordon, J., C. Davies, C. Arbeit, and M. I. Yamaner. 2023. Survey of earned doctorates. *NSF NCSES*, January 17. Available at: https://ncses.nsf.gov/pubs/nsf23300/report/postgraduation-trends (accessed May 27, 2024).

Government of Japan. 2021. *Science, technology, and innovation basic plan.* Available at: https://www8.cao.go.jp/cstp/english/sti_basic_plan.pdf (accessed May 26, 2024).

Grosse, S. D., K.V. Krueger, and J. Pike. 2018. Estimated annual and lifetime labor productivity in the United States, 2016: Implications for economic evaluations. *Journal of Medical Economics* 22(6):501–508. https://doi.org/10.1080/13696998.2018.1542520.

Gunja, M. Z., E. D. Gumas, and R. D. Williams II. 2022. The U.S. maternal mortality crisis continues to worsen: An international comparison. *The Commonwealth Fund*, December 1. Available at: https://www.commonwealthfund.org/blog/2022/us-maternal-mortality-crisis-continues-worsen-international-comparison (accessed May 25, 2024).

Gunja, M. Z., E. D. Gumas, R. Masitha, and L. C. Zephyrin. 2024. Insights into the U.S. maternal mortality crisis: An international comparison. *The Commonwealth Fund*, June 4. Available at: https://www.commonwealthfund.org/publications/issue-briefs/2024/jun/insights-us-maternal-mortality-crisis-international-comparison (accessed June 21, 2024).

Guy, J., and M. G. Peters. 2013. Liver disease in women: The influence of gender on epidemiology, natural history, and patient outcomes. *Gastroenterology & Hepatology* 9(10):633–639. Available at: https://www.ncbi.nlm.nih.gov/pmc/articles/PMC3992057 (accessed May 27, 2024).

Halbisen, A. L., and C. Y. Lu. 2023. Trends in availability of genetic tests in the United States, 2012–2022. *Journal of Personalized Medicine* 13(4):638. https://doi.org/10.3390/jpm13040638.

Haley, S. 2002. *Angel in mink: The story of Mary Lasker's crusade for medical research and the National Institutes of Health.* ACT for NIH Foundation. Available at: https://www.actfornih.org/wp-content/uploads/2023/02/Angel_in_Mink_Mary_Lasker_PDFversion.pdf (accessed May 23, 2024).

Hamel, G., and M. Zanini. 2023. America should be more like Operation Warp Speed. *The Atlantic*, December 28. Available at: https://www.theatlantic.com/ideas/archive/2023/12/operation-warp-speed-trump-lessons/676913 (accessed May 29, 2024).

Hanley, D. F., G. R. Bernard, C. H. Wilkins, H. P. Selker, J. P. Dwyer, J. M. Dean, D. K. Benjamin, Jr., S. E. Dunsmore, S. P. Waddy, K. L. Wiley, Jr., M. E. Palm, W. A. Mould, D. F. Ford, J. S. Burr, J. Huvane, K. Lane, L. Poole, T. L. Edwards, N. Kennedy, L. R. Boone, J. Bell, E. Serdoz, L. M. Byrne, and P. A. Harris. 2023. Decentralized clinical trials in the trial innovation network: Value, strategies, and lessons learned. *Journal of Clinical and Translational Science* 7(1):e170. https://doi.org/10.1017/cts.2023.597.

Harman, O., and M. R. Dietrich, eds. 2018. *Dreamers, Visionaries, and Revolutionaries in the Life Sciences.* University of Chicago Press. https://doi.org/10.7208/chicago/9780226570075.001.0001.

Heron, M. 2021. Deaths: Leading causes for 2019. *National Vital Statistics Reports* 70(9). Available at: https://www.cdc.gov/nchs/data/nvsr/nvsr70/nvsr70-09-508.pdf (accessed June 19, 2024).

Hill, L., N. Ndugga, and S. Artiga. 2023. Key data on health and health care by race and ethnicity. *Kaiser Family Foundation*, March 15. Available at: https://www.kff.org/racial-equity-and-health-policy/report/key-data-on-health-and-health-care-by-race-and-ethnicity (accessed May 24, 2024).

HIV.gov. 2023a. *Growing older with HIV.* Available at: https://www.hiv.gov/hiv-basics/living-well-with-hiv/taking-care-of-yourself/aging-with-hiv (accessed May 27, 2024).

HIV.gov. 2023b. *Impact on racial and ethnic minorities.* Available at: https://www.hiv.gov/hiv-basics/overview/data-and-trends/impact-on-racial-and-ethnic-minorities (accessed May 27, 2024).

HIV.gov. 2023c. *U.S. statistics.* Available at: https://www.hiv.gov/hiv-basics/overview/data-and-trends/statistics (accessed June 20, 2024).

HIVinfo.NIH.gov. 2023. *FDA-approved HIV medicines.* Available at: https://hivinfo.nih.gov/understanding-hiv/fact-sheets/fda-approved-hiv-medicines (accessed May 23, 2024).

Hood, L., and N. Price. 2023. *The Age of Scientific Wellness: Why the Future of Medicine Is Personalized, Predictive, Data-Rich, and in Your Hands.* Harvard University Press.

Hourihan, M. 2020. Wartime innovation: Lessons from the Office of Scientific R&D. *American Association for the Advancement of Science,* December 3. Available at: https://www.aaas.org/news/wartime-innovation-lessons-office-scientific-rd (accessed May 23, 2024).

Hoyert, D. L. 2024. Health E-stat: Maternal mortality rates in the United States, 2022. *National Center for Health Statistics Health E-Stats.* https://dx.doi.org/10.15620/cdc/152992.

IBM. 2023. Shedding light on AI bias with real world examples. *IBM,* October 16. Available at: https://www.ibm.com/blog/shedding-light-on-ai-bias-with-real-world-examples (accessed May 27, 2024).

Institute of Medicine (IOM). 2003. *Unequal Treatment: Confronting Racial and Ethnic Disparities in Health Care.* Washington, DC: The National Academies Press. https://doi.org/10.17226/10260.

IOM. 2011. *A Nationwide Framework for Surveillance of Cardiovascular and Chronic Lung Diseases.* Washington, DC: The National Academies Press. https://doi.org/10.17226/13145.

In-Q-Tel (IQT). n.d. *Home.* Available at: https://www.iqt.org/how-we-work (accessed May 27, 2024).

Investopedia. 2024. What country spends the most on research and development? *Investopedia,* March 13. Available at: https://www.investopedia.com/ask/answers/021715/what-country-spends-most-research-and-development.asp (accessed May 27, 2024).

Joint Economic Committee (JEC). 2019. *Long-term trends in deaths of despair.* SCP Report No. 4-19. Available at: https://www.jec.senate.gov/public/_cache/files/0f2d3dba-9fdc-41e5-9bd1-9c13f4204e35/jec-report-deaths-of-despair.pdf (accessed May 29, 2024).

Junod, S. W. 2007. *Statins: A success story involving FDA, academia and industry.* Available at: https://www.fda.gov/media/110452/download (accessed May 23, 2024).

Kaiser Family Foundation (KFF). 2021. The HIV/AIDS epidemic in the United States: The basics. *Kaiser Family Foundation*, June 7. Available at: https://www.kff.org/hivaids/fact-sheet/the-hivaids-epidemic-in-the-united-states-the-basics (accessed May 23, 2024).

Kandola, A. 2023. What are the most curable cancers? *Medical News Today*, March 3. Available at: https://www.medicalnewstoday.com/articles/322700 (accessed May 23, 2024).

Kauh, T. J. 2021. Racial equity will not be achieved without investing in data disaggregation. *Health Affairs Forefront.* https://doi.org/10.1377/forefront.20211123.426054.

Kennedy, B., and A. Tyson. 2023. Americans' trust in scientists, positive views of science continue to decline. *Pew Research Center*, November 14. Available at: https://www.pewresearch.org/science/2023/11/14/confidence-in-scientists-medical-scientists-and-other-groups-and-institutions-in-society (accessed May 25, 2024).

Khan, N., Z. Javed, I. Acquah, K. Hagan, M. Khan, J. Valero-Elizondo, R. Chang, U. Javed, M. B. Taha, M. J. Blaha, S. S. Virani, G. Sharma, R. Blankstein, M. Gulati, E. Mossialos, A. A. Hyder, M. Cainzos Achirica, and K. Nasir. 2024. Low educational attainment is associated with higher all-cause and cardiovascular mortality in the United States adult population. *BMC Public Health* 23:900. https://doi.org/10.1186/s12889-023-15621-y.

Khanna, G. 2021. How higher education became an important U.S. export. *Issues in Science and Technology* 38(1). Available at: https://issues.org/international-students-us-higher-education-statistics (accessed May 27, 2024).

Kington, R., S. Arnesen, W-Y. S. Chou, S. Curry, D. Lazer, and A. Villarruel. 2021. Identifying credible sources of health information in social media: Principles and attributes. *NAM Perspectives.* Discussion Paper, National Academy of Medicine, Washington, DC. https://doi.org/10.31478/202107a.

Klein, S., A. Gastaldelli, H. Yki-Järvinen, and P. E. Scherer. 2022. Why does obesity cause diabetes? *Cell Metabolism* 34(1):11–20. https://doi.org/10.1016/j.cmet.2021.12.012.

Knickman, J. R., and E. K. Snell. 2002. The 2030 problem: Caring for aging baby boomers. *Health Services Research* 37(4):849–884. https://doi.org/10.1034/j.1600-0560.2002.56.x.

Kochanek, K. D., S. L. Murphy, J. Q. Xu, and E. Arias. 2024. Mortality in the United States, 2022. *NCHS Data Brief* 492. https://dx.doi.org/10.15620/cdc:135850.

Kolata, G. 2024. First patient begins newly approved sickle cell gene therapy. *The New York Times*, May 6. Available at: https://www.nytimes.com/2024/05/06/health/sickle-cell-cure-first.html (accessed May 24, 2024).

Konstantinov, I. E. 2000. Robert H. Goetz: The surgeon who performed the first successful clinical coronary artery bypass operation. *Annals of Thoracic Surgery* 69:1966–1972. Available at: https://www.annalsthoracicsurgery.org/article/S0003-4975(00)01264-9/pdf (accessed May 23, 2024).

Kramarow, E. A., and B. Tejada-Vera. 2019. Dementia mortality in the United States, 2000–2017. *National Vital Statistics Reports* 68(2). Available at: https://www.cdc.gov/nchs/data/nvsr/nvsr68/nvsr68_02-508.pdf (accessed May 25, 2024).

Lauer, M. 2023. Trends in NIH-supported basic, translational, and clinical research: FYs 2009–2022. *NIH Extramural Nexus*, October 31. Available at: https://nexus.od.nih.gov/all/2023/10/31/trends-in-nih-supported-basic-translational-and-clinical-research-fys-2009-2022 (accessed May 24, 2024).

Lautz, A., and A. Fano. 2024. What you need to know about continuing resolutions. *Bipartisan Policy Center*, February 26. Available at: https://bipartisanpolicy.org/explainer/what-to-know-about-continuing-resolutions (accessed May 27, 2024).

Lello, L., T. G. Raben, S. Y. Yong, L. C. A. M. Tellier, and S. D. H. Hsu. 2019. Genomic prediction of 16 complex disease risks including heart attack, diabetes, breast and prostate cancer. *Scientific Reports* 9(15286). https://doi.org/10.1038/s41598-019-51258-x.

Lowder, D., K. Rizwan, C. McColl, A. Paparella, M. Ittmann, N. Mitsiades, and S. Kaochar. 2022. Racial disparities in prostate cancer: A complex interplay between socioeconomic inequities and genomics. *Cancer Letters* 531:71–82. https://doi.org/10.1016/j.canlet.2022.01.028.

Lyles, C. R., A. Aguilera, O. Nguyen, and U. Sarkar. 2022. Bridging the digital health divide: How providers and plans can help communities better adopt digital health tools. *California Health Care Foundation Issue Brief*, February. Available at: https://www.chcf.org/wp-content/uploads/2022/02/BridgingDigitalDivideProvidersPlans.pdf (accessed July 3, 2024).

Manyika, J., J. Silberg, and B. Presten. 2019. What do we do about the biases in AI? *Harvard Business Review*. Available at: https://hbr.org/2019/10/what-do-we-do-about-the-biases-in-ai (accessed May 27, 2024).

Marzban, S., M. Najafi, A. Agolli, and E. Ashrafi. 2022. Impact of patient engagement on healthcare quality: A scoping review. *Journal of Patient Experience* 9:23743735221125439. https://doi.org/10.1177/23743735221125439.

medicalcountermeasures.gov. 2024. *FDA approvals, licensures & clearances for BARDA supported products.* Available at: https://medicalcountermeasures.gov/barda/fdaapprovals (accessed May 27, 2024).

Mensah, G. A., G. S. Wei, P. D. Sorlie, L. J. Fine, Y. Rosenberg, P. G. Kaufmann, M. E. Mussolino, L. L. Hsu, E. Addou, M. M. Engelgau, and D. Gordon. 2017. Decline in cardiovascular mortality—Possible causes and implications. *Circulation Research* 120(2):366–380. https://doi.org/10.1161/CIRCRESAHA.116.309115.

Ministry of Trade and Industry Singapore. 2006. *Sustaining Innovation-Driven Growth: Science & Technology Plan 2010.* Available at: https://www.mti.gov.sg/-/media/MTI/Resources/Publications/Science-and-Technology-Plan-2010/s-and-t-plan-2010.pdf (accessed May 26, 2024).

Mitchell, C. L., A. Kennar, Y. Vasquez, K. Noris, T. Williamson, A. Mannell, A. Taylor, I. Ruberto, T. A. Cullen, M. Singeltary, S. Shah, H. Ocaranza, A. Rodriguez Lainz, and K. E. Mace. 2024. Notes from the field: Increases in imported malaria cases—Three southern U.S. border jurisdictions, 2023. *Morbidity and Mortality Weekly Report* 73(18):417419. http://dx.doi.org/10.15585/mmwr.mm7318a2.

Moses III, H., D. H. M. Matheson, S. Cairns-Smith, B. P. George, C. Palisch, and E. R. Dorsey. 2015. The anatomy of medical research: US and international comparisons. *JAMA* 313(2):174–189. https://doi.org/10.1001/jama.2014.15939.

Murphy, L. B., M. G. Cisternas, D. J. Pasta, C. G. Helmick, and E. H. Yelin. 2018. Medical expenditures and earnings losses among U.S. adults with arthritis in 2013. *Arthritis Care & Research* 70(6):811–960. https://doi.org/10.1002/acr.23425.

Murray, F. 2013. Evaluating the role of science philanthropy in American research universities. *Innovation Policy and the Economy* 13. https://doi.org/10.1086/668238.

National Academies of Sciences, Engineering, and Medicine (NASEM). 2019a. *Reproducibility and Replicability in Science.* Washington, DC: The National Academies Press. https://doi.org/10.17226/25303.

NASEM. 2019b. *Minority Serving Institutions: America's Underutilized Resource for Strengthening the STEM Workforce.* Washington, DC: The National Academies Press. https://doi.org/10.17226/25257.

NASEM. 2022. *Improving Representation in Clinical Trials and Research: Building Research Equity for Women and Underrepresented Groups.* Washington, DC: The National Academies Press. https://doi.org/10.17226/26479.

National Academy of Medicine (NAM). 2024. *Grand challenge on climate change, human health, & equity*. Available at: https://nam.edu/wp-content/uploads/2024/02/NAM-Climate-Grand-Challenge-two-pager-2.27.24.pdf (accessed May 25, 2024).

National Academy of Sciences, National Academy of Engineering, and Institute of Medicine (NAS, NAE, and IOM). 2000. *Enhancing the Postdoctoral Experience for Scientists and Engineers: A Guide for Postdoctoral Scholars, Advisers, Institutions, Funding Organizations, and Disciplinary Societies*. Washington, DC: National Academy Press. https://doi.org/10.17226/9831.

NAS, NAE, and IOM. 2007. *Rising Above the Gathering Storm: Energizing and Employing America for a Brighter Economic Future*. Washington, DC: The National Academies Press. https://doi.org/10.17226/11463.

NAS, NAE, and IOM. 2010. *Rising Above the Gathering Storm, Revisited: Rapidly Approaching Category 5*. Washington, DC: The National Academies Press. https://doi.org/10.17226/12999.

National Council on Aging (NCOA). 2023. *Get the facts on healthy aging*. Available at: https://www.ncoa.org/article/get-the-facts-on-healthy-aging (accessed July 3, 2024).

National Indian Health Board (NIHB). 2020. *Explaining Operation Warp Speed*. Available at: https://www.nihb.org/covid-19/wp-content/uploads/2020/08/Fact-sheet-operation-warp-speed.pdf (accessed May 26, 2024).

National Institutes of Health (NIH). 2015. *HIV/AIDS*. Available at: https://www.nih.gov/about-nih/what-we-do/nih-turning-discovery-into-health/hiv/aids (accessed May 23, 2024).

NIH. 2017. *Mission and goals*. Available at: https://www.nih.gov/about-nih/what-we-do/mission-goals (accessed May 28, 2024).

NIH. 2018. *NIH research planning*. Available at: https://www.nih.gov/about-nih/nih-research-planning (accessed May 25, 2024).

NIH. 2021. *To end HIV epidemic, we must address health disparities*. Available at: https://www.nih.gov/news-events/news-releases/end-hiv-epidemic-we-must-address-health-disparities (accessed May 27, 2024).

NIH. 2023a. *Spurring economic growth*. Available at: https://www.nih.gov/about-nih/what-we-do/impact-nih-research/serving-society/spurring-economic-growth (accessed May 24, 2024).

NIH. 2023b. *FY 2003–FY 2022 distribution of budget authority percentages for basic and applied research*. Available at: https://officeofbudget.od.nih.gov/pdfs/Basic%20and%20Applied%20FY%202003%20-%20FY%202022%20(V).pdf (accessed June 20, 2024).

NIH. 2024a. *Legislative chronology.* Available at: https://www.nih.gov/about-nih/what-we-do/nih-almanac/legislative-chronology (accessed May 23, 2024).

NIH. 2024b. 275 million new genetic variants identified in NIH precision medicine data. *All of Us Research Program,* February 19. Available at: https://allofus.nih.gov/news-events/announcements/275-million-new-genetic-variants-identified-nih-precision-medicine-data (accessed May 27, 2024).

NIH. 2024c. NIH to increase pay levels for pre- and postdoctoral scholars at grantee institutions. *NIH,* April 23. Available at: https://www.nih.gov/news-events/news-releases/nih-increase-pay-levels-pre-postdoctoral-scholars-grantee-institutions (accessed June 21, 2024).

NIH. n.d.a. *Selection criteria for NIH advisory committees.* Available at: https://ofacp.od.nih.gov/sites/default/files/SelectionCriteria.pdf (accessed May 29, 2024).

NIH. n.d.b. *Table #106: NIH research grants and other awards including R&D contracts—total number of awards and total and average funding by NIH Institutes/Centers and grant mechanism, fiscal years 2014–2023.* Available at: https://report.nih.gov/reportweb/web/displayreport?rId=569 (accessed June 19, 2024).

NIH Advisory Committee to the Director. 2023. *Report to the NIH Advisory Committee to the Director (ACD).* Available at: https://acd.od.nih.gov/documents/presentations/12152023_Postdoc_Working_Group_Report.pdf (accessed June 21, 2024).

National Institutes of Health, National Cancer Institute (NIH NCI). 2021. *National Cancer Act of 1971.* Available at: https://www.cancer.gov/about-nci/overview/history/national-cancer-act-1971 (accessed May 23, 2024).

NIH NCI. 2023. *Funding history.* Available at: https://maps.cancer.gov/overview/index.jsp (accessed May 25, 2024).

NIH NCI. 2024. *NCI-designated cancer centers.* Available at: https://www.cancer.gov/research/infrastructure/cancer-centers (accessed May 23, 2024).

NIH NCI. n.d.a. *The Cancer Genome Atlas Program (TCGA).* Available at: https://www.cancer.gov/ccg/research/genome-sequencing/tcga (accessed May 24, 2024).

NIH NCI. n.d.b. *Cancer Moonshot^{SM}—Recent fiscal year funding.* Available at: https://www.cancer.gov/about-nci/budget/fact-book/cancer-moonshot (accessed May 25, 2024).

NIH NCI. n.d.c. *Cancer stat facts: Cancer disparities.* Available at: https://seer.cancer.gov/statfacts/html/disparities.html (accessed May 26, 2024).

National Institutes of Health, National Center for Advancing Translational Sciences (NIH NCATS). 2024. *Community engagement across the CTSA program consortium.* Available at: https://ncats.nih.gov/research/research-activities/ctsa/projects/community-engagement (accessed May 25, 2024).

NIH NCATS. n.d. *Clinical and Translational Science Awards (CTSA) program.* Available at: https://ncats.nih.gov/research/research-activities/ctsa (accessed May 27, 2024).

National Institutes of Health, National Heart, Lung, and Blood Institute (NIH NHLBI). 2011. *Conquering cardiovascular disease.* Available at: https://www.nhlbi.nih.gov/news/2011/conquering-cardiovascular-disease (accessed May 23, 2024).

NIH NHLBI. 2024. *FY 2024 funding and operating guidelines.* Available at: https://www.nhlbi.nih.gov/current-operating-guidelines (accessed May 25, 2024).

NIH NHLBI. n.d. *Framingham Heart Study (FHS).* Available at: https://www.nhlbi.nih.gov/science/framingham-heart-study-fhs (accessed May 23, 2024).

National Institutes of Health, National Human Genome Research Institute (NIH NHGRI). 2024. *Human genome project fact sheet.* Available at: https://www.genome.gov/about-genomics/educational-resources/fact-sheets/human-genome-project (accessed May 24, 2024).

National Institutes of Health, National Institute of Allergy and Infectious Diseases (NIH NIAID). 2024. *Salary cap, stipends, & training funds.* Available at: https://www.niaid.nih.gov/grants-contracts/salary-cap-stipends (accessed May 27, 2024).

National Institutes of Health, National Institute of Arthritis and Musculoskeletal and Skin Diseases (NIH NIAMSD). 2024a. *Accelerating Medicines Partnership® rheumatoid arthritis and systemic lupus erythematosus (AMP® RA/SLE) program.* Available at: https://www.niams.nih.gov/grants-funding/funded-research/accelerating-medicines/RA-SLE (accessed May 26, 2024).

NIH NIAMSD. 2024b. *Accelerating Medicines Partnership® Autoimmune and Immune-Mediated Diseases (AMP® AIM) Program.* Available at: https://www.niams.nih.gov/grants-funding/niams-supported-research-programs/accelerating-medicines-partnership-amp (accessed May 26, 2024).

National Institutes of Health, National Institute of Diabetes and Digestive and Kidney Diseases (NIH NIDDK). 2013. *2013 award funding policy.* Available at: https://www.niddk.nih.gov/research-funding/process/award-funding-policy/2013 (accessed May 25, 2024).

NIH NIDDK. 2021. *Overweight and obesity statistics.* Available at: https://www.niddk.nih.gov/health-information/health-statistics/overweight-obesity (accessed May 25, 2024).

NIH NIDDK. 2024. *Funding trends & support of guiding principles.* Available at: https://www.niddk.nih.gov/research-funding/funded-grants-grant-history/funding-trends-support-guiding-principles (accessed May 25, 2024).

National Institutes of Health, National Institute on Drug Abuse (NIH NIDA). 2024. *Drug overdose death rates.* Available at: https://nida.nih.gov/research-topics/trends-statistics/overdose-death-rates (accessed May 25, 2024).

National Institutes of Health, National Library of Medicine (NIH NLM). 2023. *Report on the ClinicalTrials.gov modernization effort: Summary of progress: 2022–23.* Available at: https://www.nlm.nih.gov/od/bor/clinicaltrialswg/NLM_BOR_CTG_WG_Modernization_Update_Report_20231023_508.pdf (accessed May 29, 2024).

National Institutes of Health, Office of AIDS Research (NIH OAR). 2023. *NIH OAR marks 35 years of advancing HIV research.* Available at: https://www.oar.nih.gov/about/directors-corner/oar-marks-35-years-advancing-hiv-research (accessed May 23, 2024).

National Institutes of Health, Office of Budget (NIH OB). n.d. *Appropriations history by institute/center (1938 to present).* Available at: https://officeofbudget.od.nih.gov/approp_hist.html (accessed May 23, 2024).

National Institutes of Health, SEED (NIH SEED). n.d. *Product development support.* Available at: https://seed.nih.gov/product-development-support (accessed June 21, 2024).

National Postdoctoral Association (NPA). 2019. *Providing benefits for postdocs.* Available at: https://cdn.ymaws.com/www.nationalpostdoc.org/resource/resmgr/2019_launch/resources/policy/providing_benefits_for_postd.pdf (accessed June 12, 2024).

National Research Council (NRC). 2009. *21st Century Innovation Systems for Japan and the United States: Lessons from a Decade of Change: Report of a Symposium.* Washington, DC: The National Academies Press. https://doi.org/10.17226/12194.

NRC. 2014. *Convergence: Facilitating Transdisciplinary Integration of Life Sciences, Physical Sciences, Engineering, and Beyond.* Washington, DC: The National Academies Press. https://doi.org/10.17226/18722.

National Research Foundation, Prime Minister's Office Singapore. n.d. *Research, Innovation and Enterprise 2025 Plan.* Available at: https://file.go.gov.sg/rie-2025-handbook.pdf (accessed May 26, 2024).

National Science Foundation (NSF). 2018. *Definitions of research and development: An annotated compilation of official sources.* Available at: https://www.nsf.gov/statistics/randdef/rd-definitions.pdf (accessed May 28, 2024).

NSF. n.d. *75 years on the endless frontier: A vision for the future rooted in the past.* Available at: https://new.nsf.gov/science-matters/75-years-endless-frontier-vision-future-rooted (accessed May 23, 2024).

National Science Foundation, National Center for Science and Engineering Statistics (NSF NCSES). 2020a. *Survey of earned doctorates*. Available at: https://ncses.nsf.gov/pubs/nsf22300/data-tables (accessed May 27, 2024).

NSF NCSES. 2020b. *Survey of earned doctorates: Temporary visa holder plans*. Available at: https://ncses.nsf.gov/pubs/nsf22300/report/temporary-visa-holder-plans (accessed May 27, 2024).

NSF NCSES. 2021. *2021 doctorate recipients from U.S. universities*. Available at: https://ncses.nsf.gov/pubs/nsf23300 (accessed June 20, 2024).

NSF NCSES. 2022a. *Survey of graduate students and postdoctorates in science and engineering: Fall 2020*. Available at: https://ncses.nsf.gov/pubs/nsf22319#section10695 (accessed May 27, 2024).

NSF NCSES. 2022b. *Survey of Earned Doctorates (SED)*. Available at: https://ncses.nsf.gov/surveys/earned-doctorates/2022 (accessed May 27, 2024).

National Science Foundation, National Science Board (NSF NSB). 2020. *Recent trends in federal support for U.S. R&D*. Available at: https://ncses.nsf.gov/pubs/nsb20203/recent-trends-in-federal-support-for-u-s-r-d (accessed May 25, 2024).

NSF NSB. 2022. *The state of U.S. science and engineering 2022*. Available at: https://ncses.nsf.gov/pubs/nsb20221/u-s-and-global-research-and-development (accessed May 24, 2024).

Noguchi, Y. 2023a. Post-pandemic, even hospital care goes remote. *NPR*, April 29. Available at: https://www.npr.org/sections/health-shots/2023/04/29/1167392633/hospital-at-home-remote-care (accessed July 3, 2024).

Noguchi, Y. 2023b. Many generic drugs are in short supply. *NPR*, November 11. Available at: https://www.npr.org/2023/11/11/1212465756/many-generic-drugs-are-in-short-supply (accessed May 27, 2024).

Organisation for Economic Co-operation and Development (OECD). n.d.a. *Researchers*. Available at: https://www.oecd.org/en/data/indicators/researchers.html#indicator-chart (accessed July 5, 2024).

OECD. n.d.b. *OECD data explorer: Main Science and Technology Indicators (MSTI database)*. Available at: https://data-explorer.oecd.org/vis?fs[0]=Topic%2C1%7CScience%252C%20technology%20and%20innovation%23INT%23%7CResearch%20and%20development%20%28R%26D%29%23INT_RD%23&pg=0&fc=Topic&bp=true&snb=18&df[ds]=dsDisseminateFinalDMZ&df[id]=DSD_MSTI%40DF_MSTI&df[ag]=OECD.STI.STP&df[vs]=1.3&dq=.A.G%2BT_RS...&lom=LASTNPERIODS&lo=5&to[TIME_PERIOD]=false (accessed July 23, 2024).

OECD. n.d.c. *OECD data explorer.* Available at: https://data-explorer. oecd.org/vis?tm=R%26D%20expenditure%20by%20country%20 PPP&pg=0&fs[0]=Topic%2C1%7CInnovation%20and%20 technology%23INT%23%7CResearch%20and%20development%20 %28R%26D%29%23INT_RD%23&fc=Topic&snb=2&df[ds]= dsDisseminateFinalDMZ&df[id]=DSD_MSTI%40DF_MSTI&df[ag]= OECD.STI.STP&df[vs]=1.2&dq=.A.G...&pd=%2C&ly[rw]= REF_AREA&ly[cl]=TIME_PERIOD&ly[rs]=UNIT_MEASURE& to[TIME_PERIOD]=false (accessed August 1, 2024).

Otto, S. 2016. *The War on Science: Who's Waging It, Why It Matters, What We Can Do About It.* Milkweed Editions.

Park, A. 2023. U.S. HIV rates are dropping. But the progress is not equal. *Time*, May 23. Available at: https://time.com/6282076/hiv-rates-declining-us-cdc-report (accessed May 23, 2024).

Parker, E. D., J. Lin, T. Mahoney, N. Ume, G. Yang, R. A. Gabbay, N. A. ElSayed, and R. R. Bannuru. 2023. Economic costs of diabetes in the U.S. in 2022. *Diabetes Care* 47(1):26–43. https://doi.org/10.2337/dci23-0085.

Patient-Centered Outcomes Research Institute (PCORI). n.d. *Engagement tool and resource repository.* Available at: https://www.pcori.org/engagement/engagement-resources/Engagement-Tool-Resource-Repository (accessed May 25, 2024).

Peterson-KFF Health System Tracker. 2024. *How does U.S. life expectancy compare to other countries?* Available at: https://www.healthsystemtracker.org/chart-collection/u-s-life-expectancy-compare-countries (accessed May 25, 2024).

Petrullo, J. 2023. US has highest infant, maternal mortality rates despite the most health care spending. *AJMC*, January 31. Available at: https://www.ajmc. com/view/us-has-highest-infant-maternal-mortality-rates-despite-the-most-health-care-spending (accessed May 25, 2024).

PhRMA and Teconomy Partners LLC. 2022. *The economic impact of the U.S. biopharmaceutical industry: 2020 national and state estimates.* Available at: https:// phrma.org/-/media/Project/PhRMA/PhRMA-Org/PhRMA-Org/PDF/0-9/2020-Biopharma-Jobs-ImpactsMarch-2022-Release.pdf (accessed May 24, 2024).

Pryor, K., M. Barbhaiya, K. Costenbader, and C. Feldman. 2021. Disparities in lupus and lupus nephritis care and outcomes among U.S. Medicaid beneficiaries. *Rheumatic Disease Clinics of North America* 47(1):41–53. https:// doi.org/10.1016/j.rdc.2020.09.004.

Radley, D. C., J. C. Baumgartner, S. R. Collins, L. C. Zephyrin, and E. C. Schneider. 2021. *Achieving racial and ethnic equity in U.S. health care: A scorecard of state performance.* Available at: https://www.commonwealthfund.org/publications/scorecard/2021/nov/achieving-racial-ethnic-equity-us-health-care-state-performance (accessed May 27, 2024).

Read, A., and K. Wert. 2022. Broadband access still a challenge in rural affordable housing. *Pew*, December 8. Available at: https://www.pewtrusts.org/en/research-and-analysis/articles/2022/12/08/broadband-access-still-a-challenge-in-rural-affordable-housing (accessed July 3, 2024).

Research!America and Teconomy Partners, LLC. 2022. *U.S. investments in medical and health research and development 2016–2020.* Available at: https://www.researchamerica.org/wp-content/uploads/2022/09/ResearchAmerica-Investment-Report.Final_.January-2022-1.pdf (accessed May 31, 2024).

Robert Wood Johnson Foundation (RWJF). 2021. *Charting a course for an equity-centered data system: Recommendations from the National Commission to Transform Public Health Data Systems.* Available at: https://www.rwjf.org/en/insights/our-research/2021/10/charting-a-course-for-an-equity-centered-data-system.html (accessed June 21, 2024).

Rush, S., S. Uppal, C. Wang, T. Le, R. Alexandridis, L. Rice, and R. Spencer. 2021. Updated funding to lethality measures for National Cancer Institute funding allocation (2007–2017). *Gynecologic Oncology* 162(Supp 1):S322–S323. https://doi.org/10.1016/S0090-8258(21)01262-2.

Sayed, A., D. Abramov, G. C. Fonarow, M. A. Mamas, O. Kobo, J. Butler, and M. Fudim. 2024. Reversals in the decline of heart failure mortality in the US, 1999 to 2021. *JAMA Cardiology.* https://doi.org/10.1001/jamacardio.2024.0615.

Science. 2007. An Asian tiger's bold experiment. *Science* 316:38–41. https://doi.org/10.1126/science.316.5821.38

The Science Coalition. 2024. *American-made innovation sparking economic growth.* Available at: https://www.sciencecoalition.org/sparking-economic-growth/reports (accessed May 24, 2024).

Siegel, R. L., K. D. Miller, and A. Jemal. 2017. Cancer statistics, 2017. *CA: A Cancer Journal for Clinicians* 67(1):7–30. https://doi.org/10.3322/caac.21387.

Simmons-Duffin, S. 2024. How bad is maternal mortality in the U.S.? A new study says it's been overestimated. *NPR*, March 15. Available at: https://www.npr.org/sections/health-shots/2024/03/13/1238269753/maternal-mortality-overestimate-deaths-births-health-disparities (accessed July 5, 2024).

Sine, S., A. de Bruin, and K. Getz. 2021. Patient engagement initiatives in clinical trials: Recent trends and implications. *Therapeutic Innovation & Regulatory Science* 55:1059–1065. https://doi.org/10.1007/s43441-021-00306-8.

Singh, G. K., M. Siahpush, R. E. Azuine, and S. D. Williams. 2015. Widening socioeconomic and racial disparities in cardiovascular disease mortality in the United States, 1969–2013. *International Journal of Maternal and Child Health and AIDS* 3(2):106–118. Available at: https://www.ncbi.nlm.nih.gov/pmc/articles/PMC5005986 (accessed May 26, 2024).

Slingsby, B. T., and K. Kurokawa. 2013. The Global Health Innovative Technology (GHIT) Fund: Financing medical innovations for neglected populations. *The Lancet Global Health* 1(4):E184–E185. https://doi.org/10.1016/S2214-109X(13)70055-X.

Small Business Innovation Research and Small Business Technology Transfer (SBIR STTR). n.d. *Home*. Available at: https://www.sbir.gov (accessed May 27, 2024).

Smalley, E. 2018. Clinical trials go virtual, big pharma dives in. *Nature Biotechnology* 36:561–562. https://doi.org/10.1038/nbt0718-561.

Smith, K. 2023. Women's health research lacks funding—these charts show how. *Nature*, May 3. Available at: https://www.nature.com/immersive/d41586-023-01475-2/index.html (accessed May 25, 2024).

Ståhle, P., S. Ståhle, and C. Lin. 2015. Intangibles and national economic wealth—A new perspective on how they are linked. *Journal of Intellectual Capital* 16(1):20–57. Available at: https://www.stahle.fi/Intangibl_capital_and_national_economic_wealth.pdf (accessed May 24, 2024).

State Secretariat for Education, Research, and Innovation—Switzerland (SERI). n.d. *EU framework programmes for research and innovation*. Available at: https://www.sbfi.admin.ch/sbfi/en/home/research-and-innovation/international-cooperation-r-and-i/eu-framework-programmes-for-research.html (accessed May 29, 2024).

Sun, Y., and C. Cao. 2021. Planning for science: China's "grand experiment" and global implications. *Humanities & Social Sciences Communications* 8:215. https://doi.org/10.1057/s41599-021-00895-7.

Swann, J. 2018. The story behind the Orphan Drug Act. *FDA*, February 23. Available at: https://www.fda.gov/industry/fdas-rare-disease-day/story-behind-orphan-drug-act (accessed May 27, 2024).

Szabo, L. 2024. Women are less likely to die when treated by female doctors, study suggests. *NBC News*, April 22. Available at: https://www.nbcnews.com/health/health-care/women-are-less-likely-die-treated-female-doctors-study-suggests-rcna148254 (accessed July 3, 2024).

Tan, A. 2021. Record $25 billion for research and innovation over next 5 years to secure Singapore's future. *The Straits Times*, February 10. Available at: https://www.straitstimes.com/singapore/record-25-billion-for-research-and-innovation-over-next-five-years-to-secure-singapores (accessed May 26, 2024).

Temkin, S. M., E. Barr, H. Moore, J. P. Caviston, J. G. Regensteiner, and J. A. Clayton. 2023. Chronic conditions in women: The development of a National Institutes of Health framework. *BMC Womens Health* 23:162. https://doi.org/10.1186/s12905-023-02319-x.

Terrie, Y. C. 2023. Healthcare disparities in diabetes care. *U.S. Pharmacist* 48(5):37–42. Available at: https://www.uspharmacist.com/article/healthcare-disparities-in-diabetes-care (accessed May 24, 2024).

Theis, K. A., D. W. Roblin, C. G. Helmick, and R. Luo. 2018. Prevalence and causes of work disability among working-age U.S. adults, 2011–2013, NHIS. *Disability and Health Journal* 11(1):108–115. https://doi.org/10.1016/j.dhjo.2017.04.010.

Thornton, P. L., S. K. Kumanyika, E. W. Gregg, M. R. Araneta, M. L. Baskin, M. H. Chin, C. J. Crespo, M. de Groot, D. O. Garcia, D. Haire-Joshu, M. Heisler, F. Hill-Briggs, J. A. Ladapo, N. M. Lindberg, S. M. Manson, D. G. Marrero, M. E. Peek, A. E. Shields, D. F. Tate, and C. M. Mangione. 2020. New research directions on disparities in obesity and type 2 diabetes. *Annals of the New York Academy of Sciences* 1461(1):5–24. https://doi.org/10.1111/nyas.14270.

Tolbert, J., P. Drake, and A. Damico. 2023. Key facts about the uninsured population. *Kaiser Family Foundation*, December 18. Available at: https://www.kff.org/uninsured/issue-brief/key-facts-about-the-uninsured-population (accessed July 22, 2024).

Tozzi, J., R. Griffin, and S. Stein. 2020. Trump administration dips into protective gear, CDC funds to fund vaccine push. *Bloomberg*, September 23. Available at: https://www.bloomberg.com/news/articles/2020-09-23/how-much-is-the-trump-administration-spending-on-a-vaccine?embedded-checkout=true (accessed May 26, 2024).

Trapani, J., and K. Hale. 2022. *Higher education in science and engineering.* National Science Foundation National Science Board Science & Engineering Indicators. Available at: https://ncses.nsf.gov/pubs/nsb20223/international-s-e-higher-education (accessed July 3, 2024).

United for Medical Research. 2024. *NIH's role in sustaining the U.S. economy—Every state benefits.* Available at: https://www.unitedformedicalresearch.org/wp-content/uploads/2024/03/UMR-NIHs-Role-in-Sustaining-the-US-Economy-2024-Update.pdf (accessed May 24, 2024).

United Nations Enable. 2004. *"Nothing About Us, Without Us"—International Day of Disabled Persons, 2004.* Available at: https://www.un.org/esa/socdev/enable/iddp2004.htm (accessed May 25, 2024).

U.S. Environmental Protection Agency (EPA). 2024. *Climate change and human health.* Available at: https://www.epa.gov/climateimpacts/climate-change-and-human-health (accessed May 25, 2024).

U.S. Food and Drug Administration (FDA). 2019. *The history of FDA's role in preventing the spread of HIV/AIDS.* Available at: https://www.fda.gov/about-fda/fda-history-exhibits/history-fdas-role-preventing-spread-hivaids (accessed May 23, 2024).

FDA. 2023. FDA approves new medication for chronic weight management. *FDA*, November 8. Available at: https://www.fda.gov/news-events/press-announcements/fda-approves-new-medication-chronic-weight-management (accessed May 27, 2024).

U.S. Government Accountability Office (GAO). 2021. *Operation Warp Speed: Accelerated COVID-19 vaccine development status and efforts to address manufacturing challenges.* Available at: https://www.gao.gov/assets/gao-21-319.pdf (accessed May 26, 2024).

Utz, P. J., M. K. Jain, V. G. Cheung, B. K. Kobilka, R. Lefkowitz, T. Yamada, and V. J. Dzau. 2022. Translating science to medicine: The case for physician-scientists. *Science Translational Medicine.* https://doi.org/10.1126/scitranslmed.abg7852.

Valantine, H. A., and F. S. Collins. 2015. National Institutes of Health addresses the science of diversity. *Proceedings of the National Academy of Sciences* 112(40):12240–12242. https://doi.org/10.1073/pnas.1515612112.

Vlassoff, C. 2007. Gender differences in determinants and consequences of health and illness. *Journal of Health, Population and Nutrition* 25(1):47–61. Available at: https://www.ncbi.nlm.nih.gov/pmc/articles/PMC3013263 (accessed May 27, 2024).

Wagner, E., M. McGough, S. Rakshit, K. Amin, and C. Cox. 2024. How does health spending in the U.S. compare to other countries? *Peterson-KFF Health System Tracker*, January 23. Available at: https://www.healthsystemtracker.org/chart-collection/health-spending-u-s-compare-countries (accessed May 25, 2024).

Walker, M. n.d. The evolution of HIV: From death sentence to chronic condition. *MedPage Today.* Available at: https://www.medpagetoday.com/medical-journeys/hiv/106053 (accessed May 23, 2024).

Ward, Z. J., S. N. Bleich, A. L. Cradock, J. L. Barrett, C. M. Giles, C. Flax, M. W. Long, and S. L. Gortmaker. 2019. Projected U.S. state-level prevalence of adult obesity and severe obesity. *The New England Journal of Medicine* 381:2440–2450. https://doi.org/10.1056/NEJMsa190930.

Weidong, H. 2024. How Singapore punches above its weight in advancing drug discovery and development. *Agency for Science, Technology and Research Singapore*, April 19. Available at: https://www.a-star.edu.sg/News/astarNews/news/features/how-singapore-punches-above-its-weight-in-advancing-drug-discovery-and-development (accessed May 26, 2024).

Weil, D. N. 2007. Accounting for the effect of health on economic growth. *The Quarterly Journal of Economics* 122(3):1265–1306. https://doi.org/10.1162/qjec.122.3.1265.

Whellams, E. 2021. Singapore's biomedical cluster: Lessons from two decades of innovation and manufacturing policy. *Cambridge Industrial Innovation Policy*, February 19. Available at: https://www.ciip.group.cam.ac.uk/reports-and-articles/singapores-biomedical-cluster-lessons-from-two-decades-of-innovation-and-manufacturing-policy (accessed May 26, 2024).

White, D., and A. Ozimek. 2016. Healthy people, healthy economies. *Moody's Analytics*, November. Available at: https://www.bcbs.com/sites/default/files/file-attachments/press-release/201611.MoodysAnalytics.HealthPeopleHealthyEconomies.pdf (accessed May 24, 2024).

The White House. 2023. Fact Sheet: As part of President Biden's unity agenda, White House Cancer Moonshot announces new actions and commitments to end cancer as we know it. *The White House,* September 13. Available at: https://www.whitehouse.gov/briefing-room/statements-releases/2023/09/13/fact-sheet-as-part-of-president-bidens-unity-agenda-white-house-cancer-moonshot-announces-new-actions-and-commitments-to-end-cancer-as-we-know-it (accessed June 21, 2024).

The White House. 2024. OMB publishes revisions to Statistical Policy Directive No. 15: Standards for Maintaining, Collecting, and Presenting Federal Data on Race and Ethnicity. *The White House*, March 28. Available at: https://www.whitehouse.gov/omb/briefing-room/2024/03/28/omb-publishes-revisions-to-statistical-policy-directive-no-15-standards-for-maintaining-collecting-and-presenting-federal-data-on-race-and-ethnicity (accessed June 21, 2024).

Whiting, K. 2024. 6 conditions that highlight the women's health gap. *World Economic Forum*, June 19. Available at: https://www.weforum.org/agenda/2024/06/womens-health-gap-healthcare (accessed July 3, 2024).

Wieland, A., and G. T. Everson. 2018. Co-existing hepatitis C and alcoholic liver disease: A diminishing indication for liver transplantation? *Alcohol and Alcoholism* 53(2):187–192. https://doi.org/10.1093/alcalc/agx101.

World Bank. 2023. *Research and development expenditure (% of GDP)—Korea, Rep.* Available at: https://data.worldbank.org/indicator/GB.XPD.RSDV.GD.ZS?locations=KR (accessed May 27, 2024).

World Health Organization (WHO). 2020. *Life expectancy and healthy life expectancy, data by country.* Available at: https://apps.who.int/gho/data/view.main.SDG2016LEXv?lang=en (accessed May 25, 2024).

WHO. 2023a. WHO's science council issues report on mRNA vaccine technology. *World Health Organization*, December 13. Available at: https://www.who.int/news/item/13-12-2023-who-s-science-council-issues-report-on-mrna-vaccine-technology (accessed May 23, 2024).

WHO. 2023b. *Countries and territories certified malaria-free by WHO.* Available at: https://www.who.int/teams/global-malaria-programme/elimination/countries-and-territories-certified-malaria-free-by-who (accessed May 26, 2024).

WHO. 2024. *Obesity.* Available at: https://www.who.int/health-topics/obesity#tab=tab_1 (accessed May 25, 2024).

Worldometer. 2024. *COVID-19 coronavirus pandemic.* Available at: https://www.worldometers.info/coronavirus (accessed May 25, 2024).

Wouters, O. J. 2020. Lobbying expenditures and campaign contributions by the pharmaceutical and health product industry in the United States, 1999–2018. *JAMA Internal Medicine* 180(5):688–697. https://doi.org/10.1001/jamainternmed.2020.0146.

Yamaner, M. 2022. *Survey of graduate students and postdoctorates in science and engineering: Fall 2020.* National Science Foundation, National Center for Science and Engineering Statistics. Available at: https://ncses.nsf.gov/pubs/nsf22319#section10695 (accessed June 20, 2024).

Zephyrin, L. C., J. Rodriguez, and S. Rosenbaum. 2023. The case for diversity in the health professions remains powerful. *The Commonwealth Fund*, July 20. Available at: https://www.commonwealthfund.org/blog/2023/case-diversity-health-professions-remains-powerful (accessed May 27, 2024).

Zider, B. 1998. How venture capital works. *Harvard Business Review*, November–December. Available at: https://hbr.org/1998/11/how-venture-capital-works (accessed May 31, 2024).

Zippia. 2024. *Biomedical scientist demographics and statistics in the U.S.* Available at: https://www.zippia.com/biomedical-scientist-jobs/demographics/#race-statistics (accessed May 27, 2024).